Skin Sense!

Skin Sense!

A DERMATOLOGIST'S GUIDE TO SKIN AND FACIAL CARE

Stephen M. Schleicher, MD

SKIN SENSE!
A DERMATOLOGIST'S GUIDE TO SKIN AND FACIAL CARE

iUniverse books may be ordered through booksellers or by contacting:

iUniverse
1663 Liberty Drive
Bloomington, IN 47403
www.iuniverse.com
844-349-9409

ISBN: 978-1-6632-6301-8 (sc)
ISBN: 978-1-6632-6300-1 (e)

Library of Congress Control Number: 2024909877

Print information available on the last page.

iUniverse rev. date: 07/03/2024

Dedicated to the patients and staff of the
DermDox Dermatology Centers; my practice
cofounder, Dale Centofante; and the DeAngelo
family for their outstanding commitment
to patient care and our community

Contents

Introduction

Welcome to the newest edition of *Skin Sense!* and allow me to re-introduce skin, the incredibly durable outermost layer of the human body! Akin to a turtle's shell or an armadillo's plate, this essential overcoat forms a protective seal that insulates delicate structures from the environment and shields us from physical injury, temperature changes, solar radiation, harmful chemicals, and dangerous microorganisms. Yet skin not only protects but also serves to beautify. Skin is an inescapable source of our self-consciousness, attractiveness, and vanity. We often look at, touch, and caress our own skin and that of others. For those enmeshed in an image-conscious society, beauty is but skin deep. Skin mirrors and shapes our emotions: it blushes, radiates, glistens, and sweats. Skin conveys and transmits supreme pleasure and agonizing pain. We are bound by our skin, physically and psychologically.

The stamina of this remarkable tissue is incredible, given that during much of our existence, skin is tormented. Our bodies are washed daily with chemical-containing soaps and often coated with a slew of substances ranging from mass-produced cosmetics to synthetic antiperspirants. In the winter, we rush from heated, humidity-depleted buildings into subzero temperatures. In the summer, we roast under the sun's heat and penetrating rays. We dive into chlorinated pools and frolic in salt-laden oceans.

Just how enduring is skin? If the unpainted sheet-metal frame of an automobile was exposed to the same environment that confronts our body, within months, one would be left with a rusted, rotting piece of junk. Yet skin lasts a lifetime!

The key to skin's durability is its amazing regenerative power. Skin is composed of billions of living cells. As soon as one of these cells becomes injured or dies, a new one rushes to take its place. Such is the natural process of healing, and because of this biological phenomenon, any damage to our outer shell is usually temporary—usually.

As we shall see, there are times when even our skin has had enough and this updated version of *Skin Sense!* offers guidance on all facets of skin and facial care.

1

Skin Overview

OUR SKIN, THE CUTANEOUS ORGAN, IS COMPOSED OF THREE DISTINCT layers: the epidermis, the dermis, and subcutaneous (or fat) tissue. The following brief description of each layer will aid in the understanding of both healthy and diseased skin.

The epidermis is our outermost coating and the one visible to our eyes. It is the thinnest of all layers; over much of the body, the depth is only one-sixteenth of an inch thick, as thick as this page. The epidermis is thickest on the palms and soles, where it may reach nearly one-eighth of an inch.

The epidermis contains both living and dead cells. New cells are produced in the lowest portion, the basal layer. These cells migrate upward to the surface and become the cornified layer. Here the cells form a resilient, waterproof material known as keratin. Dead surface cells are continuously shed as miniscule flakes (scales) and are immediately replaced by living cells from the layers below. Some twenty-eight days are required for a new cell produced in the basal layer to finally reach the outer cornified zone; in other words, complete replacement of the epidermis takes nearly one month.

The epidermis is devoid of blood vessels. This alone gives some indication of the thinness of this layer, as we all have experienced bleeding following a superficial nick or cut. Even the most trivial of wounds easily traverse the thin epidermis to enter the next layer, the dermis.

The dermis is some forty times thicker than the epidermis. Besides harboring blood vessels, it also contains nerves, sweat glands, and sebaceous oil glands. The dermis feeds the cells of the basal layer and regulates growth of the entire epidermis. The tautness of the skin is in large part due to the collagen and elastin fibers that reside in the dermis.

The dermis rests on a thick pad of fat called the subcutaneous layer. This layer, like the epidermis, varies in thickness, depending on body location. It is practically nonexistent within the eyelid and, as you might guess, becomes thickest around the waist. The subcutaneous tissue serves as a thermal insulator and shock absorber.

Unhealthy skin may result from a disease process that affects any of the three layers. For example, dry skin involves changes in the epidermis, acne is a disorder of sebaceous glands located in the dermis, and cellulite arises from alterations in the subcutaneous tissue.

MALE AND FEMALE SKIN

Is male skin from Mars and female skin from Venus? Hopefully, we are all earthlings, but differences in the sexes certainly carry over to our skin as well. Male skin is thicker than female skin. Increased collagen and elastin fibers in men contribute to firmness and are a reason why men tend to age with fewer deep-set wrinkles and fine lines than women. A greater number of hair follicles also contributes to aging disparity. Over time, exposure to solar radiation breaks down dermal collagen; facial hair (the male beard) acts as a physical screen to ultraviolet light.

Male skin has more active oil and sweat-gland activity than female skin; thus, men have less need to moisturize. Bacteria living on the skin surface degrade sweat, resulting in the characteristic musty aroma of the male armpit and the enhanced need for deodorants (at least when out in public).

The placement of fat is to some degree sex-related and varies in males and females. The distribution in women gives rise to the more rounded contours associated with the feminine figure and contributes to culturally defined attractiveness.

BLACK AND WHITE SKIN

Pigment cells within the skin are called melanocytes, and the actual pigment is known as melanin. Melanin production varies among various cultural groups, such as Africans, Asians, and Caucasians. Interestingly, black skin does not contain more melanocytes, but it does contain more melanin. The melanin granules are larger and darker.

Variations in human skin color have evolved over the ages. Black skin is the most resistant to ultraviolet light and is ideally suited to withstand chronic sun exposure. Indeed, unprotected white or pale skin is a sitting duck for skin cancer.

A redeeming feature of sunlight is that it induces production of vitamin D, which is important for our health and well-being. Here melanin serves as a double-edged sword. By blocking solar radiation, melanin protects against skin cancer, but it also inhibits vitamin D production.

2

Nutrition and the Skin

THREE MAIN FOOD TYPES ARE CARBOHYDRATES, PROTEINS, AND FATS, all of which contribute in various ways to healthy skin.

Despite occasional pitches to the contrary, a true superskin diet does not exist. Perhaps one day what we eat will serve as a fountain of youth that thwarts the aging process. For now, one would do best to follow the sound nutritional principles that medical doctors advocate for much of the population: a diet low in calories, high in fiber and whole grains, and moderate in saturated fats, with reduced levels of salt and sugar.

The role of diet in causing or perpetuating our most common skin conditions is somewhat controversial. A diet rich in fat does not make the skin oilier, and drinking large amounts of fluid will not put moisture back into the skin. Does chocolate worsen breakouts? Possibly. Recent data suggests that eating refined carbohydrates and sugar leads to a surge in an insulin-like growth factor that triggers an excess of male hormones. Male hormones signal skin cells to excrete sebum (oil). Increased sebum production is a contributing factor to pimple formation.

An allergic reaction to a particular food or food additive may result in hives. Common offenders include strawberries and shellfish. One uncommon skin disease, called dermatitis herpetiformis, is linked to gluten sensitivity. Gluten is found in many foods, including bread and beer.

Marked fluctuations in weight may also affect the skin. Gaining pounds augments the amount of body fat, which in turn predisposes a person to stretch marks and cellulite. Rapid weight loss (from crash dieting,

4

for example) may result in decreased skin turgor and a worsening of the appearance of cellulite.

Vitamins and minerals are substances found in our food and in our home cabinets required for proper maintenance of the body. Botanicals are compounds that contain extracts or active ingredients derived from plants. Nutraceuticals are products that have been isolated or purified from food and are used for medicinal purposes. Vitamins, minerals, botanicals, and nutraceuticals may be ingested or applied topically to the skin. Note that the labeling of an herbal or botanical product as *natural* or *organic* means nothing regarding efficacy. The fact that something comes from a plant does *not* make it safe or effective. Examples include tobacco and poison ivy.

To follow is a review of many commonly encountered vitamins, minerals, botanicals, and nutraceuticals. Separating reality from hype is not an easy task.

ACAI

Acai, a berry cultivated in Central and South America, contains potent antioxidants and is a rich source of the flavonoid anthocyanin, which is purported to protect the skin from free radicals and inhibit the aging process. Taken orally, acai is said to have cardioprotective, anticancer, and antidiabetic beneficial effects. Topical compounds are limited in concentration due to the propensity for skin staining, and to date, solid clinical studies documenting efficacy are lacking.

ALPHA LIPOIC ACID

Alpha lipoic acid (ALA) is a potent antioxidant that helps to deactivate free radicals. It also has anti-inflammatory activity. ALA is found in only trace amounts in food. Oral supplementation has been used as treatment for diabetic neuropathy and Alzheimer's disease.

Topical preparations contain ALA in concentrations ranging from 1 percent to 5 percent. ALA is readily absorbed through the skin and can enter the dermis and subcutaneous layers. Small studies demonstrated positive results when ALA was used to minimize wrinkles and decrease sun-induced pigmentation.

ALOE VERA

Aloe vera is one of the most widely used botanical products. The gel is found within the leaves of the aloe vera plant and consists of 99.5 percent water and a collection of polysaccharides. Aloe vera has been reported to increase blood flow, reduce inflammation, and promote healing, and it has been used to treat many skin diseases, including eczema, psoriasis, and even genital herpes. Aloe is found in hundreds of over-the-counter preparations, including moisturizers, soaps, sunscreens, and shampoos, but many contain concentrations so low that any therapeutic effect from this plant is dubious. Despite the widespread consumer use of aloe, there is a paucity of high-quality scientific research documenting its effectiveness other than as a run-of-the-mill moisturizer. One study concluded that aloe vera applied to burns did not speed healing of skin.

BIOTIN

Biotin is a water-soluble B vitamin necessary for metabolism and growth. The compound is found in many foods, including liver, soy products, carrots, and cereals. Deficiency is rare and, curiously, may be induced by a diet rich in raw eggs, as a substance in egg whites prevents intestinal absorption of the vitamin. The first signs of biotin deficiency involve the hair and nails, which lose luster and become brittle. So will taking excess biotin in pill form strengthen these integuments? The evidence to date is not convincing. Further, in 2017, the FDA issued a warning cautioning on the harmful effects of high-dose biotin. According to the FDA, "biotin in blood or other samples taken from patients who are ingesting high levels of biotin in dietary supplements can cause clinically significant incorrect lab test results. The FDA has seen an increase in the number of reported adverse events, including one death, related to biotin interference with lab tests." Advise your health-care provider if you are taking biotin supplements.

CANNABIDIOL

Cannabidiol (CBD) is an active ingredient in cannabis, and use in skincare products is trending after the US government legalized certain hemp-derived products in 2018. Research indicates these plant-derived substances have anti-inflammatory, analgesic, and anti-itch properties. Small clinical trials have demonstrated improvement of various conditions, including acne, arthritis, eczema, psoriasis, and scars, although overall effectiveness awaits the outcome of larger studies.

COENZYME Q10

Coenzyme Q10, also called ubiquinone-10, is a cellular antioxidant found in all tissues of the body, including skin. This vitamin-like substance is abundant in organ meats, such as heart, liver, and kidney, as well as in soybean oil and certain fish. Oral supplementation has been used as an adjunct to cancer therapy and in the management of Parkinson's disease and congestive heart failure.

Coenzyme Q10 is now found in a variety of lotions and creams and is claimed to have antiaging effects. The skin levels of this compound decrease naturally with age, and a small study demonstrated a beneficial effect on wrinkles about the eye.

COFFEEBERRY EXTRACT

Coffeeberry, derived from the crushed, processed fruit of the *Coffea arabica* plant, is another trendy antioxidant utilized in creams and is purported to promote skin rejuvenation, limit environmental damage, and lighten pigmentation. Taken orally, coffeeberry prevented exercise-induced oxidative stress during training periods and, in high doses, enhanced brain function.

COCONUT OIL

Coconut oil is another trending so-called superfood and one that contains a high level of short- and medium-chained saturated fats. The benefit of these substances on the cardiovascular system is highly contested, and several organizations, including the American Heart Association, recommend consuming them in moderation. One study demonstrated that topically applied coconut oil improved eczema in pediatric patients with mild to moderate disease.

GRAPE SEED EXTRACT

Grape seed extracts contain an ample supply of polyphenols. Although some are like those found in tea, others have distinct properties. Scientific data supports the antioxidant activities of these compounds, which are said to be more potent than vitamins C and E. Applied topically, grape seed extracts are claimed to improve skin tone, prevent scars and stretch marks, hasten wound healing, and protect against sun damage. More clinical studies are needed to support such claims. Resveratrol is a potent antioxidant found in the skin of red grapes and red wine, which—in massive doses—may or may not prevent or reduce the ravages of cellular aging. Studies in mice are promising. However, meaningful long-term safety and efficacy data are several years away. Stay tuned.

GROWTH FACTORS

Growth factors are a group of proteins that play a role in wound healing and tissue regeneration. Growth factors incorporated into skin creams and serums may come from a variety of sources, including cell cultures, placental cells, and plants. Kinetin is a plant-derived growth factor that has antioxidant properties and retards the aging of certain cells. Kinetin lotions are, in general, nonirritating. Preliminary studies indicate that like retinoids, growth factors may improve wrinkles and dark spots. However, skin cells do contain retinoid receptors but not kinetin receptors, leaving the efficacy of this product in doubt.

HYALURONIC ACID

Hyaluronic acid is a naturally occurring glycosaminoglycan. In the skin, this substance contributes to elasticity and hydration. With age, the concentration diminishes, resulting in skin dryness and laxity. This sugar-based compound is added to creams and topical serums to increase fullness and decrease water loss. Several dermal fillers contain hyaluronic acid, which is injected under the skin to correct wrinkles and depressions. The beneficial effect is immediate.

LECITHIN AND PHOSPHATIDYLCHOLINE

Lecithin and its purified derivative, phosphatidylcholine, are components of cell membranes. Choline, the major constituent of phosphatidylcholine, is found naturally in soybeans, oatmeal, liver, cabbage, and cauliflower. Several skin-care formulations contain lecithin, which is used primarily for its moisturizing properties. A liquid form of phosphatidylcholine is a component of mesotherapy, an injection technique used to absorb fat cells. This drug is not approved for use in the United States, and the safety and efficacy of this procedure have not been satisfactorily documented.

LYCOPENE

Lycopene is an antioxidant found in high concentration in red tomatoes (including juice, sauce, paste, and ketchup). The substance concentrates in certain organs, including the prostate gland, colon, and skin. High intake of food substances containing lycopene is associated with a decreased risk of gastrointestinal and prostate cancer. Lycopene and related compounds (called carotenoids) may help protect the skin from ultraviolet light damage, and several commercially available creams incorporate this compound in conjunction with other vitamins. Claims that such products will boost collagen production or reduce wrinkles and crow's-feet have not been substantiated.

NICOTINAMIDE

Nicotinamide (or niacinamide) is a derivative of niacin, a component of the B vitamin complex. These compounds enable our cells to produce energy and also help repair damage to DNA induced by sun exposure. A deficiency of this vitamin is rare but leads to the condition known as pellagra, which is characterized by dementia and a skin rash. B vitamins are found in a variety of plant and animal food sources.

Application of nicotinamide to the skin may help prevent moisture loss and sun damage. Some data indicates that topical niacinamide has anti-inflammatory properties and may improve acne and rosacea. Oral nicotinamide supplementation may protect against solar radiation and reduce formation of pre–skin cancers (actinic keratoses) and skin cancers.

PEPTIDES

Peptides are compounds containing amino acids, which serve as the building blocks of proteins, such as collagen. A few appear to aid in the healing of ulcers and wounds and are thought to do so by stimulating collagen production. Results of small industry-sponsored studies using a variety of peptides (some containing copper) demonstrate improvement of wrinkles and photoaging, and several facial lotions and eye creams containing peptides are on the market.

PYCNOGENOL

Pycnogenol is an extract made from the bark of French maritime pine. The compound contains flavonoids and is claimed to prevent cardiovascular disease and decrease leg swelling when taken orally. Pycnogenol is an antioxidant and is incorporated into several skin creams, some of which claim sun-protection, skin-lightening, and antiaging properties. There is a dearth of scientific evidence supporting such claims.

SOY PROTEINS

Soybeans contain ingredients called flavonoids that are structurally related to the female hormone estrogen. Women with high dietary intake appear to have lessened risks of breast cancer and cardiovascular disease. Studies in mice demonstrate that topically applied soy protein protects against ultraviolet light and decreases the occurrence of skin cancer. Soy proteins also show promise as skin-lightening and collagen-stimulating agents.

TEA EXTRACTS

Green tea, black tea, and oolong tea contain substances called polyphenols, which have significant antioxidant and anti-inflammatory activity. In animals and humans, the application of a green-tea ointment appears to lessen the incidence of ultraviolet-induced skin cancers, and tea-derived polyphenols are now found in several skin-care formulations. Antiwrinkle and skin-smoothing claims have also been made. Determination of the true benefit of topically applied tea extracts awaits the outcome of larger clinical studies.

TURMERIC

Turmeric is a spice commonly used in Asian and Indian foods. The biologically active component, curcumin, has documented anti-inflammatory properties. Topical application studies support facilitation of wound healing and the prevention of skin cancer. Worldwide, especially in India, curcumin is often added to skin-care preparations.

VITAMIN A

Vitamin A is a fat-soluble vitamin that plays an important role in maintaining healthy skin. The substance is found in certain food items, such as eggs, whole milk, and liver, and it is added to fat-free milk and many cereals. Retinol is an active form of the vitamin, and beta-carotene (found in leafy green vegetables) is a vitamin A precursor.

In the United States, vitamin A deficiency is a rare occurrence. An excess of this vitamin is usually the result of dietary supplement overindulgence. Because vitamin A is fat-soluble, it can be stored in the body and can accumulate in harmful levels. Too much vitamin A can damage the liver and may contribute to osteoporosis. Signs of acute toxicity include nausea, vomiting, headache, and visual disturbances. Pregnant women should avoid vitamin A supplementation since the substance is a known teratogen (inducer of birth defects).

Topical and oral vitamin A–based compounds are used to treat acne. The FDA-approved derivatives tazarotene and tretinoin may diminish fine lines and wrinkles. The vitamin A compounds retinol and retinyl palmitate are found in over-the-counter products, and these too may improve the appearance of aging skin. Clinical trials comparing the efficacy of the prescription versus nonprescription topical formulations are still lacking.

VITAMIN C

Vitamin C (ascorbic acid) is a water-soluble vitamin that plays a key role in the formation of collagen, a substance necessary for healthy bones, cartilage, muscle, and blood vessels. This vitamin is acquired mostly by eating fruits and vegetables, and healthy individuals who eat balanced diets rarely need supplementation. Vitamin C deficiency (extraordinarily rare in the United States) leads to a condition called scurvy, which is characterized by joint pains, muscle weakness, gum bleeding, and skin lesions. Except for gastric irritation, oral intake of large amounts of the vitamin does not appear to have serious consequences, nor does it appear to have much benefit, despite at one time being touted as a cure for the common cold and a preventative of cancer.

Of late, vitamin C has been incorporated into a variety of over-the-counter preparations touting antiaging and anti-inflammatory properties. Vitamin C is a powerful antioxidant that may, when used topically, stimulate collagen production and offer some level of protection against the damaging effects of sunlight. The problem is that vitamin C in topical formulations is highly unstable and rapidly breaks down when exposed to the environment (which is why most products are packaged in dark containers). More documentation of the stability, skin-penetrating abilities, and efficacy of currently marketed products is needed before they can be recommended from a therapeutic standpoint. Vitamin C products are well tolerated, and many are formulated within elegant, moisturizing bases.

VITAMIN D

Vitamin D is a hot topic, as a significant percentage of elderly Americans are deficient in this vitamin, and low levels are linked to osteoporosis and, less convincingly, to heart disease and cancer. The body uses this vitamin to regulate bone development and maintenance. The Institute of Medicine recommends that adults receive 600 IU (international units) of vitamin D daily, and those above age seventy should receive 800 IU. The Endocrine Society recommends higher doses and states that most adults can safely take between 1,000 and 2,000 IU daily. Toxicity from too much vitamin D is uncommon but can manifest as fatigue, weakness, dehydration, and constipation. Vitamin D is found in fortified milk; fatty fish, such as salmon; and dietary supplements. It is also produced in the skin upon exposure to sun and ultraviolet light, hence the name *sunshine vitamin*. Lighter skin produces more vitamin D than darker skin. Just five to ten minutes outdoors three times weekly allows many individuals to produce the necessary amount of this vitamin. However, dietary supplementation is recommended for those who cannot tolerate the sun, have a family or personal history of skin cancer, lack access to sunlight, are elderly, or have darker complexions. Routine screening of adults for vitamin D deficiency is controversial, and unfortunately, supplementation does not reduce fractures or prevent cancer in healthy adults. That said, a Harvard study found a reduced incidence of rheumatoid arthritis and psoriasis in adults taking 2,000 IU of vitamin D daily for five years,

VITAMIN E

Vitamin E is a fat-soluble vitamin found naturally in vegetable oils, nuts, and leafy green vegetables. Deficiency of this vitamin is rare, and the merits of supplementation are contested. Indeed, vitamin E is an example of the hype associated with antioxidants and the aging process. Thirty years ago, this vitamin was trumpeted as a retardant of cell death, helping to gobble up damaging free radicals, the harmful by-products of metabolism and sun exposure. Megadoses were in vogue. No longer. The American Heart Association warns that high doses of vitamin E may increase the risk of bleeding and stroke, and other studies find no evidence of cancer prevention. Further, one study demonstrated that men taking high-dose vitamin E supplements doubled their risk of prostate cancer.

Vitamin E has been used for decades as an ingredient in certain over-the-counter treatments for dry skin and, more recently, for its postulated antiaging properties. Topical vitamin E (in the form of either alpha tocopherol or tocopherol acetate) has antioxidant properties, which, in animal models, protect epidermal cells from environmental damage, such as that caused by sunlight. To date, human studies are inconclusive, perhaps in part because this vitamin, like vitamin C, has difficulty penetrating the skin.

VITAMIN K

Vitamin K is a fat-soluble vitamin that helps to activate the clotting mechanism of blood. This vitamin is found in cabbage and leafy green vegetables, such as spinach and soybeans. Deficiency of this vitamin results from diseases that interfere with intestinal absorption but is rare.

Several topical formulations contain vitamin K and claim to reduce the severity of bruising, diminish the appearance of tiny leg veins, and even improve dark circles under the eyes. Very little scientific data substantiates any of these claims, although one small study using topical vitamin K reported diminished bruising following laser treatment for facial blood vessels.

ZINC

Zinc is an essential mineral that has diverse physiological functions and plays a critical role with enzymes and proteins needed to maintain healthy skin. It is found in abundance in beef, pork, lamb, and peanuts. Dietary deficiency of zinc is very unusual in the United States. Certain rare genetic disorders are caused by the inability to absorb zinc, resulting in inflamed skin and rashes. Zinc has anti-inflammatory and antibacterial properties and is incorporated into shampoos to control dandruff. Topical zinc oxide

Stephen M. Schleicher, MD

is used as a skin protectant and sunscreen. Oral zinc supplementation has been reported to improve acne, although evidence of a beneficial effect is far from convincing. In doses greater than forty milligrams per day, zinc can be toxic, and supplementation has been linked to an increased risk of advanced prostate cancer as well as to reduced levels of HDL ("good") cholesterol.

3

Dry Skin

PROBLEMS ASSOCIATED WITH DRY SKIN RANK AMONG THE MOST COMMON complaints fielded by dermatologists. Consumers spend more than $300 million each year on over-the-counter preparations used to alleviate the annoying manifestations of moisture-depleted skin. Dry skin (also called xerosis) is the result of excessive water loss from the outermost layer of the epidermis, the stratum corneum. Signs of this condition become apparent when skin water loss interferes with the normal flexibility of this organ. Dry skin is characterized by roughness, chafing, cracking, and, in more severe cases, redness and inflammation.

The moisture content of the stratum corneum is in large part responsible for the normal appearance of skin. Hydration of this top layer is impacted by the relative humidity and temperature of surrounding air. Rapid evaporation of water readily occurs in cold weather and at low humidity. For this reason, dry skin is most common during the winter months. Air-conditioning and forced-air heating also promote skin dryness. As the skin loses moisture, tiny cracks appear on its surface, which is the initial stage of skin chafing.

Placing the skin in contact with water will not add moisture to the outer layer. In fact, this may have the opposite effect. Too-frequent bathing is a common contributing factor to dry skin. The body coats its surface with a protective mixture of sweat and oils produced by specialized glands in the dermis to help minimize environmental damage. Frequent washing, especially with harsh detergent soaps, removes this protection and causes the skin to dry out at an accelerated rate. Showering or sitting in the tub more than once a day is discouraged for those afflicted with dry skin. And it's best to use lukewarm water, as hot water tends to be even more drying.

One might assume that drinking ample fluids replenishes the moisture content of skin. This advice is frequently recommended by health and beauty magazine columnists. It's not true. Drinking five or six glasses of water a day is good for the kidneys but will not rehydrate the epidermis of a nondehydrated human.

Moisturizers are the most effective means both to minimize and to treat xerosis. Lubricating creams, lotions, and ointments form a semiocclusive film over the skin's surface, minimizing evaporative water loss. Emollients are agents that fill in spaces between skin cells, soothing rough skin. Ingredients with emollient properties include lanolin, butyl stearate, and petrolatum. Emollients are either water- or oil-based. In general, water-based moisturizers are easier to apply and do not clog facial pores, whereas oil-based compounds are more occlusive and more effective in preventing water loss from the skin surface. Some moisturizers deposit substances called humectants on the skin surface; these agents facilitate water absorption. Examples of humectants include lactic acid, urea, and glycerin. Compounds that help repair and restore skin-barrier function include ceramides, stearic acid, and palmitic acid. Individuals with sensitive skin should avoid fragranced formulations, and those anticipating sun exposure should use moisturizers with sunscreen.

Commonsense measures to minimize dry skin include avoidance of frequent washing and harsh soaps; instead, substitute lubricating cleansers specially formulated for sensitive skin. Add bath oil to every bath. After leaving the bath or shower, apply a moisturizer while the skin is still damp to trap a thin film of water on the skin's surface. Moisturize frequently, and in cold weather, modify the environment by using a humidifier. Adhering to these simple procedures will help improve skin that is dry, rough, scaly, and flaky.

4

Itchy Skin

ITCHING (MEDICALLY TERMED *PRURITUS*) IS A SENSATION THAT PRODUCES a desire to scratch. We itch because our skin has itch-sensitive nerve endings termed *pruriceptors*. Itching may be localized to a specific area (for example, the site of a mosquito bite), or it may be generalized over the entire skin surface. People respond to an itch in different ways, with the response in part depending upon the persona of the affected individual. A mosquito bite, for example, may be violently scratched until it bleeds, gently rubbed, or simply ignored.

A wide range of factors can induce itching. These include inflammations of the skin caused by external irritants, such as harsh soaps; infections (especially those caused by yeast and fungi); infestations, such as scabies and lice; allergic reactions, including contact dermatitis and hives; and specific skin disorders, such as eczema.

Generalized itchiness may be associated with internal conditions requiring medical attention. Diabetes, liver disease, kidney failure, and even cancer are, at times, accompanied by diffuse itching. Itchy skin may also occur during pregnancy.

A very common cause of itching is dry skin (xerosis). Too-frequent bathing with hot water and strong soaps, advanced age, and cold weather all contribute to skin dryness. The legs are the most commonly involved sites. The condition may be improved with moisturizing creams and bath oils.

An often-overlooked source of itching is psychological overlay. An anxious male may scratch his scrotum; the back of the neck is a common location in females.

People suffering from psychosis may believe their skin has been invaded by parasites or fibers. Afflicted individuals pick and dig until sores develop. Terms used to describe such behavior are *delusions of parasitosis* and *Morgellons disease.*

Itching can be a distressing symptom. Itch is made worse by wool clothing, friction, excess warmth and sweating, reduction of body oils by frequent washing, and the use of harsh soaps. Inactivity tends to make one more aware of an itch; hence, itching is usually most severe at night.

A self-limited itch, such as an insect bite or a mild case of poison ivy, may be lessened by cool compresses and application of over-the-counter anti-itch preparations. Chronic conditions associated with itching and skin findings, such as eczema, are best addressed by a dermatologist. Generalized itchiness may require a medical and laboratory workup to rule out an internal medical condition.

PRURITUS ANI

Anal itching (pruritus ani) is a common, annoying problem. The condition may be triggered by numerous factors, including anxiety; hemorrhoids; contact with irritating chemicals and soaps; parasites (crabs, lice, and pinworms); and fungal and yeast infections. Circumstances that worsen the itching include excess perspiration, obesity, tight clothing, frequent bowel movements, inadequate cleansing, and occupations that require long periods of sitting (for example, truck driving or office work).

Several general measures may provide total or partial relief of pruritus ani. Cleansing after each bowel movement should be particularly thorough, using only minimal amounts of a mild, nonmedicated soap. All soap must be completely rinsed off the area after cleansing. Moistened facial tissue, rather than ordinary toilet tissue, causes less irritation. Prolonged sitting (during long car trips, for example), tight clothing, and overstuffed chairs should be avoided. A daily sitz bath and frequent applications of an occlusive paste, such as zinc oxide ointment, may prove beneficial. Cases of pruritus ani that do not respond to these measures should be evaluated by a dermatologist, gynecologist, or proctologist.

5

Aging and the Skin

THE SKIN IS NO DIFFERENT FROM ANY OTHER ORGAN IN THE BODY; IT too ages. But unlike other organs, aging skin is visible to us and to others.

Young skin is characteristically taut, smooth, and evenly pigmented. Skin that is old has become thin, discolored, lax, and wrinkled. As skin ages, several distinct changes occur. Aged skin suffers from fluid depletion. The water-holding capacity diminishes, and the oil-secreting glands dry up. This often results in dryness, chapping, and scaling.

Physiologic functions of skin include barrier protection, temperature regulation, sweat production, sensation perception, and production of vitamin D. By middle age, many of these functions are reduced, some by as much as 50 percent or more. Senile skin is characterized by a thinning out of the outermost layer, the epidermis. In some elderly people, the skin becomes so atrophic that it resembles cigarette paper.

The layers under the epidermis—the dermis and the subcutaneous tissues—also decrease in thickness. Tiny fibers that support the skin lose their springiness; when stretched, the skin of an older person does not bounce back, as would the skin of a young person. As skin matures, collagen becomes fragmented, and new production is reduced. The combination of tissue loss coupled with loss of elasticity results in the hallmark of aged skin: wrinkles.

Aged skin is more susceptible to a variety of disorders and diseases than normal skin. Because of the lack of moisture, senile skin has a tendency to dry out. This is especially severe in low humidity. As skin dries, it becomes chapped, cracked, and intensely itchy. The more aged the skin, the greater the number of dilated and broken blood vessels. Skin cancer occurs at an accelerated rate with each passing year. Besides cosmetic disfigurement, this problem poses a real threat to general health.

Three main factors are known to contribute to skin aging: heredity, sunlight, and smoking.

Much of the aging process is genetically determined, programmed into an individual's body even before birth. The process is termed *intrinsic aging* or *chronological aging*. If your parents have young-looking skin, chances are good that barring physical abuse, you will too. Unfortunately, the contrary also holds true. The skin of some individuals seems to age at an advanced rate no matter how much it is pampered.

The rare condition called progeria is characterized by premature aging of all organs, including the skin. Children with this disease have wrinkled, aged skin comparable to the skin of an elderly individual. Werner syndrome is a similar-appearing condition that becomes evident in the late teens. The genetic defects responsible for both disorders have been identified and, hopefully, will shed additional light on the normal aging process.

The sun is a bitter enemy of healthy skin. Repeated, prolonged exposure to sunlight leads to irreversible premature aging, called photoaging. Ultraviolet light stimulates formation of free radicals that damage DNA and decrease the amount of collagen in the dermis. Excessive sunlight leads to thinned and yellowed skin, broken blood vessels, brownish discolorations (liver spots), and skin cancer.

One can appreciate the injurious effects of sunlight by examining the skin of a person who has spent a great deal of time outdoors. Look closely at the face of an inveterate fiftyish-year-old sun worshipper. That person most likely appears much older due to premature skin aging. Indeed, if you are one who has spent much time in sunlight, compare the skin of your face and hands to that of your buttocks and, if female, the underside of your breasts. The areas exposed to chronic sun are apt to be discolored, rough, and wrinkled. That beautiful tan of yesteryear has long ago faded, leaving in its wake damaged, unhealthy skin.

Several studies document that cigarette smoking leads to premature aging of the skin. One study comparing identical twins found that the skin of the twin who smoked was 25 percent thinner than that of the twin who did not. On a molecular level, cigarette smoke activates genes responsible for a skin enzyme that breaks down collagen.

The term *smoker's face* was coined more than two decades ago by a physician who was able to differentiate smokers from nonsmokers not by the soot and carcinogens clogging their lungs but by facial features alone. The smoker's face is characterized by accelerated skin aging, deep wrinkles about the mouth, and accentuated crow's-feet. Even secondhand smoke is absorbed through the skin.

Regarding premature aging, we cannot alter our genes. But we can in large measure control exposure to sunlight and cigarette smoke.

DERMATOLOGICAL TREATMENT OF THE AGING FACE

Few enjoy the aging process, especially when it involves the skin. Given that we cannot turn back the hands of time, what can we do to reverse the ravages of aging?

Topical Antiaging Compounds

Several prescription drugs known as retinoids may help delay the aging process: Refissa (identical to Retin-A, which is used to treat acne) and Avage (identical to Tazorac, also used to treat acne) are FDA approved to help minimize fine wrinkles and mottled hyperpigmentation. These medications work, albeit slowly and when used in tandem with sun protection. Note that neither will work on deeper wrinkles or creases.

When applying a retinoid, use only a miniscule amount to avoid undue dryness and irritation. A pea-sized amount is enough to cover the entire face. A good regimen is to apply a moisturizer with sunscreen in the morning and apply the prescription antiaging medication at night.

A number of nonprescription skin creams are widely available and heavily promoted. Active ingredients include retinol (a form of vitamin A), vitamin C serums, various peptides, resveratrol, and alpha hydroxyl acids.

Microdermabrasion

Microdermabrasion is a cosmetic procedure that uses a vacuum-suction device to exfoliate surface skin cells. Most commonly, fine aluminum oxide crystals are applied to the face via a wand. A diamond-tipped head may also be used. The treatment is popular in spas and dermatologist offices and does not require medical supervision. Dead skin cells are literally sucked away from the epidermis. Skin rejuvenation changes are subtle. Repeat treatments may stimulate new collagen formulation.

Chemical Peels

Chemical peels have been used to rejuvenate facial skin for decades. Peeling involves the application of an exfoliating or wounding agent to the surface of the skin. Depth of penetration and degrees of exfoliation and skin sloughing are dependent on a number of factors, with the most important being the chemical used for the peel. Other factors may include concentration of the peeling agent and time left on the skin surface.

A light peel stimulates epidermal rejuvenation by gently removing the stratum corneum. A medium-depth peel causes partial destruction of the epidermis and induces inflammation. Deep peels are uncommonly utilized, because of the risk of scarring and pigment alteration.

Superficial peels are used to improve the tone and texture of skin. Commonly used peeling agents are glycolic and salicylic acids. Side effects are minimal and include transient dryness and redness.

Medium-depth peeling agents include Jessner's solution, glycolic acid, and low to medium concentrations of trichloroacetic acid. These may even texture and tone, lighten dark spots, and diminish fine lines secondary to sun damage. Redness is to be expected, which fades over a seven- to ten-day period. Complications include untoward pigmentary changes (especially in people with dark skin), reactivation of fever blisters, and (rarely) scarring. Chemical peels may be combined with laser resurfacing for facial rejuvenation.

Botox, Daxxify, Dysport, and Xeomin

Botox was approved for cosmetic use in 2002 and soon became the most widely performed cosmetic procedure in the United States, with millions of injections administered yearly. The simplicity of administration, rapidity of results, lack of serious side effects, and high degree of satisfaction combined to revolutionize the field of minimally invasive aesthetic procedures. Botox is a so-called neurotoxin and now competes with similar agents that include Daxxify, Dysport, and Xeomin.

Neurotoxins are most commonly used to temporarily correct forehead creases, frown lines, and wrinkles about the eyes (crow's-feet). Administered through a tiny needle, the entire procedure takes minutes and entails minimal discomfort. Visible results are noted within days after injection. The effect lasts three to four months on average, somewhat longer with Daxxify. Off-label, neurotoxins are used about the mouth ("lip flip") and even on neck muscles. The cost of neurotoxins varies. Some providers charge based on areas treated; others charge by the amount (units) administered.

Neurotoxin side effects are uncommon and include headache and eyelid drooping. The latter, medically termed *ptosis*, is a temporary but disconcerting nuisance that may last anywhere from a few days to a few weeks. Upneeq eye drops may improve ptosis.

In 2009, the FDA added a black-box warning of possible serious side effects related to use of neurotoxins. Given the millions of injections and the rarity of adverse events, it appears that serious reactions have occurred only as a result of off-label use for certain chronic disease states, not for the treatment of wrinkles and lines. Nevertheless, finding a well-trained, experienced health-care provider to administer the neurotoxin is always a wise decision.

Dermal Fillers

Although neurotoxins are very effective in minimizing forehead lines and crow's-feet, they cannot restore fullness, particularly to the mid and lower face. Indeed, volume loss is one of the hallmarks of an aging face, and dermal fillers are ideally suited for this purpose.

The first dermal fillers approved by the FDA were made from bovine (cow) collagen. Collagen is one of the foundations of the dermis. Products were short-lived and could trigger allergic reactions, necessitating allergy testing prior to use.

Fat transplantation bypasses the need for allergy testing, since injected fat is taken from the abdomen or backside of the same individual. A major drawback is longevity, as not all transplanted cells survive the procedure. Injecting platelet-rich plasma (PRP) simultaneously may enhance survival. Commonly treated areas are the cheek hollows, nasal folds, undereye bags, and hollows of the eyes.

The dermal filler market exploded in 2003 with FDA approval of Restylane. Restylane is non-animal-derived hyaluronic acid, a normal component of the body substance that surrounds skin cells. Prior allergy testing is not required, which allows for same-day administration. Repeated injections may stimulate the natural production of collagen. The Restylane line now includes Restylane Silk, Restylane Lyft, Restylane Refyne, Restylane Defyne, Restylane Kysse, and Restylane Contour. Nearly thirty additional FDA-approved hyaluronic acid fillers are available, including Belotero; Juvederm (Ultra, Voluma, Volbella, Vollure); Revanesse Versa; and the RHA collection (RHA 2, RHA 3, and RHA 4). Correction lasts for several months to more than a year. Side effects include redness, bruising, and persistent bumps. If bumps persist, these can be dissolved with the

27

injectable enzyme hyaluronidase. Rare side effects include skin breakdown (necrosis) and vision loss.

Radiesse is a filler composed of calcium. This product has no allergic potential, and the correction often lasts eight months or longer. Radiesse augments existing collagen and stimulates production of new collagen as well. This product may be diluted with saline, which decreases thickness. Sculptra consists of poly-L-lactic acid and is not a conventional replacement filler. Small amounts are injected over time, and the end result is stimulation of collagen. Visible results are gradual and develop over weeks. Bellafill is an injectable collagen filler with microspheres that provides both immediate and longer-term correction.

As a rule, the longer a filler lasts, the more careful (and experienced) a provider should be in administering it. The choice of filler often depends on the area to be treated.

Nasolabial folds (the two creases running from the nose to the corners of the mouth) and marionette lines (creases from the mouth corners to the chin) are amenable to most fillers. Factors to consider are price, longevity, and the experience and preference of the medical provider performing the injections. Lip augmentation requires a less viscous filler to avoid the complication of persistent bumps. Corrections about the eye and temple entail minute amounts of a thinner filler, whereas depressions of the midcheek region are best handled with a thicker volumizer or dermal stimulator.

Laser Rejuvenation

Laser resurfacing is characterized as either ablative or nonablative. Ablative resurfacing entails wounding of the skin surface. Lasers for this purpose are the CO2 and erbium:YAG varieties. During the ablative process, the epidermis and parts of the dermis are removed, which results in improvement of skin texture, evening of pigmentation, and some correction of wrinkles. Downtime is significant, with marked redness and crusting lasting at least ten days. Scarring is possible, and the procedure is best not performed on more darkly pigmented individuals. Fractional ablative lasers break light into thousands of microbeams that bore tiny holes in the epidermis. The result is skin tightening of variable degree with less downtime. Healing occurs within six to ten days.

With nonablative resurfacing, the beam of laser light passes through the epidermis to stimulate new collagen production in the dermis. Downtime is nil, with minimal redness. The results are often subtle and may not become apparent for weeks to months. A series of treatments are required approximately four to eight weeks apart. Periodic touch-ups are recommended.

Intense pulsed light (IPL) uses nonlaser light to improve pigmentation, reduce unsightly blood vessels, and smooth texture. This too is a nonablative technique.

Nonablative fractional resurfacing utilizes a laser to create so-called micro–thermal zones of controlled skin damage. Mildly photodamaged skin usually improves with this technique, but deeper wrinkles do not.

Antiaging is a big business. Looking one's best can often be accomplished with minimal discomfort and virtually no downtime. The use of neurotoxins, dermal fillers, volumizers, and lasers will continue to soar.

6

The Sun and Skin

A SUBSET OF OUR SOCIETY REVERES THE SUN, WITH BRONZED SKIN A symbol of leisure and good health. Soaking up rays is often a favorite pastime, and come nightfall, a glance in the mirror reveals the payoff of a day's work: the suntan.

WARNING: SUN EXPOSURE MAY BE HAZARDOUS TO YOUR HEALTH

Some may express concern about the hazards of nuclear power yet think nothing of basking all day in solar radiation. The sun's ultraviolet rays damage the skin's elastic tissues, leading to unsightly skin lines, discolorations, wrinkles, and, for some, skin cancer. Each year, more than two million cases of skin cancer are diagnosed in the United States. Ultraviolet light is responsible for the majority of these cancers.

Besides the long-term effects attributed to chronic sun exposure, the damage wrought by sunlight may become apparent much sooner. Acute overexposure results in the painful, all-too-familiar sunburn.

SUNBURN

Virtually every light-skinned person has experienced sunburn at one time or another. Sunburn is a discomforting condition most frequently encountered at the beginning of summer, before a tan has been acquired. Redheads and blonds burn readily; dark-skinned persons may sunburn but require more prolonged exposure to strong sunlight. A study of fifteen thousand adults found that one-third had experienced a sunburn within the past year.

The extent of sunburn may range from a mild, painless redness to an exquisitely tender, blistering fiery-red eruption. A mild burn begins some six to twelve hours from the beginning of exposure, reaches a maximum redness within twenty-four hours, and gradually declines over the next few days, leaving in its wake tanned skin that may take more than one week to reach its peak.

Severe sunburn also begins six to twelve hours following sun exposure, but within one to two days, marked skin changes occur. Skin becomes extremely painful to even the slightest sensation. Chills, fever, and nausea are commonplace. Fluid-filled blisters appear, and layers of the skin begin to slough off. Uneven pigmentation and even scarring may result.

Mild sunburn reactions may be treated with cool water compresses. Emollient creams can soothe the skin and relieve dryness. Over-the-counter burn preparations contain local anesthetics that may help alleviate discomfort but will not enhance healing. Aspirin controls the pain and may lessen the inflammation.

Severe sunburn should be treated by a physician. Cortisone pills and antibiotic creams are sometimes necessary to limit inflammation and prevent infection.

SUN PROTECTION: HOW TO REMAIN SAFE IN THE SUN

Six different skin types are defined based on skin pigmentation. The lower the skin type number, the greater the risk of developing significant damage from exposure to sunlight or indoor tanning.

Skin, Sunburn, and Tanning Type Traits

1. Sensitive: Always burns easily; never tans
2. Sensitive: Always burns easily; tans minimally
3. Normal: Burns moderately; tans gradually
4. Normal: Burns minimally; always tans well
5. Insensitive: Rarely burns; tans profusely
6. Insensitive: Never burns; deeply pigmented

The sunlight that reaches the earth consists of visible light and ultraviolet (UV) radiation; the invisible ultraviolet rays cause suntan and sun-induced skin injuries. The amount of ultraviolet light reaching the skin depends on several factors. For example, the lower the latitude, the greater the risk of sun damage to the skin at any given hour. A noontime sunbather in Miami will experience a heavier dose of burning rays than a noontime sunbather in Boston. The time of greatest risk anywhere in the world occurs in the middle of summer between the hours of 10:00 a.m. and 2:00 p.m.

Seasonal variations and altitude also play a role in the amount of ultraviolet light striking the skin. Given the same time and duration of sun exposure, one will experience a more severe suntan in early May than at the end of August. The higher the altitude, the less atmosphere is present to filter out ultraviolet rays. This is a contributing factor to the sunburns often seen in winter skiers.

Environmental factors may amplify the likelihood of sunburn. Beach sand, snow, and shiny metal (as in sun reflectors) increase the dose of solar radiation impacting the skin. And other modalities may fail to offer adequate protection. Water is not an efficient sun blocker, and burning rays can penetrate beneath the surface of a pool. As for cloud cover, one can still sunburn on overcast days. Seventy percent of the sun's rays penetrate clouds and fog.

Potentially harmful ultraviolet radiation is divided into UVA and UVB. UVA constitutes more than 90 percent of the radiation penetrating to the earth's surface. UVA can also penetrate the skin's surface and has been implicated in suppression of the immune system and causation of skin cancer. UVB causes damage to the epidermis, resulting in acute sunburn. Chronic ultraviolet light exposure induces wrinkles and other signs of cutaneous aging. UVB is filtered by window glass, but UVA is not.

A first line of defense against untoward ultraviolet light exposure is clothing, with some garments much more effective than others. Certain clothes, especially when wet, fail to protect the skin from a significant portion of ultraviolet light. Color (with darker shades being more efficient), fiber content, and fabric weave help determine clothing's effectiveness as a barrier to ultraviolet light.

Individuals who are extremely sun-sensitive and at high risk for skin cancer may consider specially formulated protective clothing when sun avoidance is not possible. Manufacturers include Coolibar and Solumbra. Another option is to wash clothes using the laundry additive Rit SunGuard, which confers adequate UV light protection that lasts for about twenty washes.

And don't forget a hat, especially if your hair is thinning. The hat protects not only the scalp but also, depending on brim size, parts of the face.

Sun protective agents applied to the skin are known as sunscreens. These are formulated as creams, gels, lotions, sticks, pads, and sprays. Some ingredients work best to block UVA and have esoteric names, such as avobenzone (Parsol 1789) and terephthalylidene dicamphor sulfonic acid (Mexoryl SX). Others block UVB and have equally unpronounceable names, including octyl dimethyl para-aminobenzoic acid (PABA) and ethylhexyl p-methoxycinnamate. Agents that block both UVA and UVB are referred to as inorganic sunscreens and contain titanium dioxide or zinc oxide.

Since both the ultraviolet A and ultraviolet B spectrums of light are dangerous to skin, one should always apply a sunscreen labeled *broad spectrum*.

For maximum effectiveness, sunscreens should be applied thirty minutes before sun exposure and reapplied after swimming or profuse sweating. As a rule, most sunscreens lose their effectiveness after three or four hours. A water-resistant sunscreen will adhere to the skin while the user is in water for forty minutes. A very-water-resistant sunscreen will adhere for eighty minutes. No sunscreen can make the claim it's waterproof.

The amount of sunscreen applied is an important factor. One ounce (two tablespoons) is the minimum amount needed to cover the entire body. According to a study published in the *British Journal of Dermatology*, most people only apply one-quarter of the amount of sunscreen they should.

Concerned about the growing incidence of sun-related skin problems, as well as undocumented claims by several manufacturers, the US Food and Drug Administration advised in 1978 that sun protection factor rating (SPF) must be included on all sunscreen packages. Sunscreen products carry numbers ranging from 15 to 50-plus, indicating their effectiveness in filtering out solar radiation capable of burning the skin.

The higher the SPF number, the greater the shielding from burning radiation. This is not a linear relationship; an SPF of 30 does not give twice as much sun protection as an SPF of 15. SPF 15 blocks 93 percent of burning rays, SPF 30 blocks 97 percent, and SPF 50 blocks all but 1 percent. In 2013, the FDA mandated that any product with an SPF lower than 15 must carry a label warning that it will not protect against skin cancer. The FDA also questions the merit of using any sunscreen labeled above 50.

Remember, SPF refers *only* to UVB radiation protection. Maximum sunscreen protection is afforded by a high-SPF, broad-spectrum formulation. This is important because UVA radiation has been linked to premature aging and skin cancer. And again, applying the correct amount of sunscreen is crucial. Using half of the correct amount of sunscreen rated at SPF 50 (that is, one tablespoon rather than two) will not give a SPF of 25 but one of 8. Given that most people apply an inadequate amount of sunscreen, one study suggests that many consumers use an SPF 100 over an SPF 50 for maximum protection.

When used properly, sunscreens will prevent the immediate danger from solar radiation, the sunburn. Long-term use will help prevent wrinkles, dark spots, and cancer. Because the hazardous effects of sunlight are cumulative, sunscreens are best used at an early age.

KIDS AND SUNSCREEN

Sunscreens are not recommended for children younger than six months; regardless of age, small tots are best physically shielded from direct sunlight. The FDA is investigating the use of spray-on sunscreens due to the risk of particle inhalation and exacerbation of asthma or allergic reactions. It is best for children to avoid sprays. Several sunscreens are specifically marketed for children, and these contain ingredients less likely to irritate the skin, such as titanium dioxide and zinc oxide.

INDOOR TANNING

The Food and Drug Administration and the American Academy of Dermatology are very concerned about the health hazards posed by indoor tanning centers. You should be as well. Sunbed ultraviolet light emission is ten times more potent than natural sunlight. Most of the radiation received in tanning booths is ultraviolet A, linked to skin cancers and cataracts. Because of these risks, the majority of states have enacted age restrictions regarding light-box tanning, and some now prohibit the use of indoor tanning booths by minors. In 2014, the FDA mandated that all indoor tanning devices carry warning labels. Still, some thirty million Americans are expected to tan indoors annually. In one study, about 20 percent of high school girls and 5 percent of high school boys had sought out some form of indoor tanning at least once in the previous year.

Melanoma is the second most common cancer among American women in their twenties, and the rate of new melanoma cases in younger women has soared, increasing by 50 percent since 1980. Women under thirty-five who use sunbeds increase their risk of developing melanoma by an astounding 74 percent. Melanoma has the potential to kill.

The Department of Health and Human Services and the World Health Organization have deemed ultraviolet light a known carcinogen (cancer-promoting agent). The number of skin cancer cases due to indoor tanning is higher than the number of lung cancer cases due to smoking.

A review in the *Journal of the American Academy of Dermatology* offers an apt summary: "Evidence demonstrates unequivocally that tanning beds cause sunburn, photoaging, development of skin cancer, and full addictive behaviors while supplying no scientifically supported health benefits."

TANOREXIA

The concept that UV tanning is addictive has gained ground over the past several years, and the condition has been given the name *tanorexia*. Studies have demonstrated that some frequent tanners experience withdrawal symptoms when UV tanning is abruptly discontinued. A study of college students found that 12 percent of those interviewed showed evidence of a UV light-substance-related disorder. Despite awareness of the dangers of tanning, many are of the notion that tanner people are better-looking and healthier.

SELF-TANNERS

Scores of self-tanning formulations are available for those seeking to *look* tan. The first self-tanning product was introduced back in 1960, Coppertone QT (Quick Tanning) lotion. The problem? Rather than looking golden brown, users tended to resemble aged pumpkins. Fortunately, shades are now quite realistic and pleasing. This fact, coupled with increased public awareness of the dangers of ultraviolet light, has contributed to the rising popularity of self-tanning products.

The most effective sunless tanning gels, lotions, and sprays contain an ingredient called dihydroxyacetone (DHA), a colorless sugar that stains

36

the cells in the top layer of the epidermis. DHA is the only agent currently approved by the FDA for this purpose. Stained cells are already dead and slough off in about five to seven days, hence the need for reapplication. Many commercial products contain a mixture of DHA, bronzers (water-soluble dyes that temporarily stain skin), and moisturizers. DHA appears to be safe long-term when used on the skin surface, with low incidence of allergic reactions. Keep in mind that most products containing DHA offer no—or, at best, inadequate—sun protection, and stained skin remains vulnerable to ultraviolet damage. Note as well that the FDA discourages the use of indoor tan spraying.

Tan accelerators are said to lessen the exposure time needed to bronze skin. Many contain the amino acid tyrosine, and all require ultraviolet light for activation. The FDA is "not aware of any data demonstrating that tyrosine or its derivatives are effective in stimulating the production of melanin." (Stimulation of melanin is what produces a suntan.)

Oral tanning pills often contain the substance canthaxanthin, which is FDA approved as a food-coloring agent. In high quantities, the compound is deposited in the skin. But it is also deposited in the liver and eyes and can lead to hepatitis and cataracts. Canthaxanthin as a tanning agent is now banned in the United States but is available via the internet. People are also searching the web for the hormone melatonin-2, a tanning stimulator that is incorporated into nasal spray. This substance has been linked to new mole formation and possible melanoma.

SAD

No doubt, when the sun doesn't shine, many of us become depressed. This is termed SAD (*seasonal affective disorder*), and its features are depression, lack of energy, and an increased need for sleep. The mildest form is known by most as *winter blues*. About 75 percent of those affected are women, and the most common age of onset is in the midthirties. SAD is believed to affect fifteen million Americans. The treatment of choice is bright light—the visible kind—not ultraviolet. And the light does no good by only striking the skin; it must be visualized by the eye.

MORE ON VITAMIN D

Vitamin D helps the body absorb calcium and maintain adequate levels of this mineral in the bloodstream; both tasks are necessary for the maintenance of healthy bones. Vitamin D is the most commonly supplemented vitamin, added to milk, bread, and orange juice. Sunlight induces skin cells to manufacture vitamin D. The amount produced depends on a number of factors, including exposure time, altitude, latitude, extent of skin surface exposed, time of year, and skin pigmentation (the darker or more tanned the skin is, the less is produced). Use of a high-SPF sunscreen limits or even prevents the skin from forming vitamin D.

Vitamin D deficiency can lead to bone diseases, including osteoporosis. Some research suggests that higher levels of vitamin D may protect against prostate, colorectal, and breast cancers. However, many people do not obtain the minimum amount of this vitamin. By advocating strict sun protection to avoid skin cancer, are doctors limiting an important source of this very important vitamin?

Studies document that relatively small amounts of sun exposure—ten to fifteen minutes on sunscreen-free hands, face, and arms two to three times a week—are sufficient to maintain adequate levels. So a little sun should go a long way.

Yes, a little sun. Millions of dollars each year are spent on topical formulations and procedures to prevent or reverse the ravages of aging. Yet a major factor that contributes to the aging process is sun and ultraviolet light exposure. And yes, some individuals can tolerate ample sun exposure, especially those with darker skin. Others cannot. Individuals of skin type

38

one (persons with very pale skin, blue eyes, and blond or red hair) and skin type two (persons with fair skin) experience skin damage with each and every exposure. If you keep smoking cigarettes, the chances are pretty good that you will develop lung cancer or emphysema. If you keep chasing a golden tan, the day may soon arrive when that taut, bronzed, "healthy" covering gives rise to a shriveled, discolored, cancer-plagued prune.

7

Social Media and Looks

SOCIAL MEDIA PLATFORMS, SUCH AS FACEBOOK, INSTAGRAM, TIKTOK, YouTube, and X, attract a global audience and influence the lives of countless individuals. One benefit is immediate access to medical advice from both health-care professionals and fellow patients. A recent study revealed that at least one in five Americans turns to these platforms prior to seeking medical consultation. That is all well and good, except when this information is incorrect or, worse, dangerous. One study found that more than 60 percent of dermatology content shared on social media was either wrong or misleading.

Social media consumption by impressionable teenagers and adults plays a significant role in causing or exacerbating body dissatisfaction. Preoccupation with looks permeates this media. When advising on skin conditions or look enhancement, many influencers have no formal dermatology background and promote products or routines that lack clinical study. One example is acne. An online study of individuals with acne found that nearly 50 percent of participants used social media as a base for acne treatment, with women accounting for 75 percent of this population. Unsurprisingly, many online recommendations did not follow established guidelines. Another study of popular TikTok and Instagram posts dealing with hair loss revealed that most were created not by medical specialists but by nonmedical influencers and wig companies.

Dangerous social media trends related to appearance can ricochet across the internet. *Looksmaxing*, a term applied to self-betterment, shows no sign of abating. Several of these trending lifestyle modifications have the potential to harm. Already discussed is melatonin-2, which is claimed not only to stimulate tanning but also to induce weight loss and enhance sexual performance. Nicknamed the *Barbie drug*, this hormone is snorted into the nose, is not regulated by the FDA, and has potential for serious long-term side effects.

Another trend that defies belief is face smashing. Impressionable and misguided male teenagers are convinced that fracturing their facial bones will lead to a movie actor's chiseled look. Bone-smashing videos have more than 250 million views.

By enhancing and updating our knowledge and awareness of health and beauty, social media conveys priceless benefits to society. Far from priceless is the amplification of falsehoods, charlatans, and abject stupidity that this media encourages and perpetuates.

8

Disorders of Pigment

VITILIGO

VITILIGO IS A COMMON SKIN DISORDER THAT AFFECTS MORE THAN TWO million persons in the United States. The condition manifests as one or more white spots devoid of pigment on the skin. The depigmentation may appear anywhere on the body. Most cases begin before the age of twenty years, and more than 70 percent will have occurred by age thirty.

Vitiligo may remain stationary for years or may rapidly progress to involve a large portion of the skin surface. Areas of vitiligo produce no symptoms; however, because of the lack of pigment, painful sunburn readily develops with even brief sun exposure. Vitiligo is often of great cosmetic concern. The darker the original skin color, the more noticeable the condition. The psychological effects may be devastating. More than one-half of all persons with vitiligo admit that the condition has significantly impaired the ability to interact with others socially. Seeking advice from a mental health counselor or vitiligo support group is encouraged. One such group is the American Vitiligo Research Foundation (avrf.org).

Vitiligo therapy is not universally successful. Specialized light treatments (narrow-band UVB, excimer laser, and PUVA) have been a mainstay of therapy for years and require multiple therapy sessions. Early vitiligo may respond to application of potent topical steroids, such as clobetasol or the calcineurin inhibitors Elidel (pimecrolimus) and Protopic (tacrolimus). In 2022, the topical JAK inhibitor Opzelura (ruxolitinib) became the first prescription medication approved to treat vitiligo. This cream is applied twice daily to affected areas. Oral JAK inhibitors are awaiting approval as well. Individuals with vitiligo should always use a broad-spectrum sunscreen on affected areas; this will help protect the skin from becoming sunburned and from developing skin cancer.

Visible sites of pigment loss can be concealed with pigmented cover-ups, such as Covermark and Dermablend. Lighter-skinned individuals may benefit from the application of self-tanning agents containing dihydroxyacetone. An option for severe vitiligo is permanent depigmentation with the topical bleaching agent monobenzone. This is a drastic step, as the loss of pigment is irreversible and permanent. The process can take from one to four years. Michael Jackson is believed to have undergone such therapy.

MELASMA

Melasma is a condition that presents as mottled brownish patches on the face. The most common sites are the cheeks, nasal bridge, forehead, and skin above the upper lip. The condition invariably affects women and is most common in darker-skinned ethnic groups, such as Asians, Indians, and Hispanics. Melasma is believed to affect some six million women in the United States.

Several factors play a role in the development of melasma, including a hereditary predisposition. Hormonal changes are also implicated. Melasma occurring in pregnant females is referred to as *chloasma* ("the mask of pregnancy"). Melasma may be induced or worsened by both birth control pills and exposure to sunlight.

Treatment of melasma may prove challenging. If the condition is related to pregnancy, gradual resolution may follow delivery. If the condition began while on oral contraceptives, discontinuation of the pill is often deemed advisable.

Protection from ultraviolet light is essential, including sun avoidance and sun protection utilizing daily application of a broad-spectrum sunscreen, the higher the SPF the better. This is important, as window glass does not block out ultraviolet radiation of the A range.

Some cases of melasma will respond to a combination of sun protection and topical application of the bleaching agent hydroquinone. Hydroquinone inhibits an enzyme responsible for the production of melanin. The FDA removed over-the-counter bleach creams from the US market in 2020, citing the potential for untoward pigmentary changes attributed to misuse. Higher concentrations (greater than 2 percent) are available by prescription.

Tri-Luma or similar compounded agents are effective topical therapies. These prescription creams combine hydroquinone, a topical steroid, and tretinoin. Azelaic acid (Azelex, Finacea), tazarotene (Tazorac), adapalene (Differin), and glycolic acids also have skin-lightening properties. No matter which agent is chosen, response is slow, requiring a minimum of three months of therapy. Microdermabrasion may enhance the efficacy of topical agents. Lasers and chemical peels can prove of value but may, on occasion, stimulate increased pigmentation. Oral tranexamic acid is a promising therapeutic option. This medication is approved by the FDA but not for this indication. Caution is advised because of the possible risk of blood clots.

AGE SPOTS

Many individuals develop unsightly, flat dark spots on sun-exposed areas, especially the face and hands. Called *liver spots* by some, these have nothing to do with the liver. The spots are medically benign but cosmetically unsightly. Additional darkening may be prevented by sun avoidance and use of broad-spectrum sunscreens. The lesions often respond to liquid nitrogen cryosurgery and laser treatment. The topical bleaching agents described above are of limited use. Many brightening products are marketed with ingredients such as niacinamide, bearberries, soy, licorice extract, vitamin C, kojic acid, and oligopeptide-34. Some are pricey—and of questionable efficacy—but are probably safer than hydroquinone for long-term use.

9

Benign Skin Growths

BENIGN GROWTHS ARE SKIN LESIONS THAT ARE NOT CANCEROUS (malignant). They may be annoying from a cosmetic standpoint, but they do not endanger one's overall health.

SKIN TAGS

Skin tags are tiny, soft, fleshy outgrowths of skin that usually have an onset in early to middle adult life. They more frequently occur in women and are found around the neck, upper chest, and armpits. The color ranges from flesh-colored to light brown.

Skin tags cause no discomfort or itching unless irritated. They can be removed by careful snipping with a pair of manicure scissors. Larger tags are best treated in the doctor's office.

SEBORRHEIC KERATOSIS

Have you ever noticed, on many beaches, seniors dotted with darkly colored, seemingly stuck-on growths? These unsightly lesions are known as seborrheic keratoses.

Seborrheic keratoses are most common after the age of fifty. They are almost always multiple and range in color from yellow to brown to dark black. The surface texture may feel waxy or rough. Common locations are the chest and back, but they may also occur on the face, scalp, and extremities. An individual lesion may attain a size of two or more inches in length, and they can become irritated by friction or trauma.

Seborrheic keratoses are benign skin growths that do not turn into skin cancers. They are prone to irritation and are readily removed in a dermatologist's office either by minor surgery or by freezing with liquid nitrogen.

BIRTHMARKS AND MOLES (NEVI)

Birthmarks and moles are lesions composed of specialized pigment cells. One can consider a mole to be a birthmark that arises on the skin's surface later in life. The term *nevus* is applied to both entities.

Nevi are common, and many persons have more than a dozen. Some nevi may be present at birth, but the majority arise in young adulthood. Many flat moles tend to fade away with advancing age.

Nevi come in a variety of different sizes, shapes, and colors. They range in size from pinpoint specks to expansive lesions covering a large part of the body. Coloration runs the spectrum from flesh-colored to blue, tan, and even pitch black. Some are perfectly flat, while others are elevated and dome-shaped. Their surface may be smooth or rough, and some may even have hair.

Most nevi are best left alone. Some occur in areas where they are easily traumatized or cosmetically unacceptable, and these can be removed simply. Rarely, a mole may turn into a potentially lethal skin cancer (melanoma), and for this reason, nevi should be checked on a periodic basis. The following changes warrant immediate evaluation by a dermatologist:

1. any rapid increase in size;
2. any changes in coloration, especially red or whitish hues;
3. the development of notched, irregular borders;
4. the onset of itching; or
5. the onset of spontaneous bleeding.

All persons with a family history of melanoma or a history of sunburn should have their skin examined on a regular basis.

WARTS

Warts are common skin growths caused by a virus. The infection occurs most frequently in children, and the sites usually affected are the fingers, hands, and soles of the feet.

Since warts are caused by a virus, they are contagious. Warts may be spread to different parts of the body as well as to other persons. Many individuals are apparently immune and do not develop warts even when exposed to them.

Warts are classified into several subtypes:

- *Common Wart.* The common wart is familiar to virtually everyone. This growth appears as a rough-surfaced, flesh-toned-to-brown skin projection that slowly enlarges in size. The sites most often involved are the hands and fingers. The appearance of one wart may be followed in several weeks by one, two, or numerous other warts.
- *Plantar Wart.* This wart grows on the bottom of the feet and resembles a callus. It occurs on the weight-bearing areas of the sole and may become painful.
- *Flat Wart.* These flesh-colored warts are small, smooth, and slightly raised. Flat warts may occur on the face
- *Genital Wart.* The genital wart presents as a flesh-colored-to-pinkish-red growth in the vaginal or anal regions or as a firm projection on the shaft of the penis. As with other forms, these growths are spread by close personal contact, in this case by sexual relations. For this reason, genital warts are considered a sexually transmitted disease (STD). More than five hundred thousand new cases are diagnosed each year.

Warts are often bothersome from a cosmetic standpoint. Fortunately, about two-thirds disappear without any therapy within two years. Oddly, psychological coaxing (for example, hypnotic suggestion) may result in rapid clearance. This is possibly the reason why folk remedies, such as burying a potato under a stump or rubbing a copper penny over the wart, were reported to cure the condition. Topical salicylic anti-wart solutions, gels, and patches can be purchased without prescription at any pharmacy. Warts may also be treated in the doctor's office by cryosurgery, electric needle (electrodessication), or laser. Most dermatologists prefer to use liquid nitrogen (cryosurgery) because the procedure is effective, is rapidly performed, and does not involve injection of a local anesthetic. Plantar warts often prove difficult to destroy. Care must be taken to avoid aggressive surgical treatment, as painful scarring may result.

Genital warts are treated with liquid nitrogen cryosurgery, electrodessication, acid solution, or application of a substance called podophyllin. Imiquimod cream (Aldara) and podofilox gel (Condylox) are prescription at-home therapies for genital warts.

Genital warts are directly linked to the development of cervical cancer. Women potentially exposed to the virus are urged to have Pap smears performed on a regular basis. Strains of genital warts (HPV) may also cause oral, anal, and penile malignancies. A vaccine (Gardasil 9) protecting against these strains is effective and widely available. The Centers for Disease Control (CDC) recommends that all preteens receive the HPV vaccination, which may be given as early as age nine years and is best administered before a person is sexually active. This is the first time a vaccine has been documented to prevent cancer.

CALLUSES AND CORNS

A callus is an area of thickened skin that appears over sites of repeated or prolonged friction and pressure. The area involved is yellow and roughened.

Calluses are most commonly located on the palms and serve as a clue to the activity of a person—for example, the callused hands of a bowler or tennis player.

A corn is a discomforting, raised area of skin with a smooth, firm surface that produces pain on pressure. Corns arise most frequently on the top and sides of the fifth toes. Tight, poorly fitting shoes are the usual cause.

Corns and calluses may be treated with acid plaster applied to the lesion and covered with adhesive tape. Painful corns may require surgical removal. Wide, well-fitting shoes prevent the recurrence of most corns.

10

Premalignant Growths and Skin Cancer

EACH YEAR, MORE THAN TWO MILLION NEW CASES OF SKIN CANCER are diagnosed in the United States, and the number is steadily increasing. Skin cancers account for more than half of all malignancies, and one in six Americans will develop skin cancer in his or her lifetime. Advanced skin cancer can lead to tissue destruction, disfigurement, and even death.

Sun exposure is a major contributing factor to the development of skin cancer. Ninety percent of these tumors occur on body sites often unprotected from solar radiation—that is, on the face, ears, neck, and hands. Persons who have spent a great deal of time outdoors, such as fishermen, gardeners, and lifeguards, are at greatest risk. The incidence of skin cancer is highest in areas receiving large amounts of ultraviolet radiation; persons living in Miami or Phoenix have a two to three times greater chance of developing skin cancer than persons living in Chicago or New York.

Heredity too plays a role in the development of skin cancer. Those with fair skin and light eyes (for example, persons of Nordic, Irish, or British descent) are at greater risk than persons with darker pigmentation. Persons who redden and blister readily increase their risk of skin cancer with each prolonged exposure to sunlight.

PRECANCEROUS LESIONS

A precancerous lesion is one that has the potential to evolve into a true cancer. Three major types of precancerous lesions exist: solar keratosis, leukoplakia, and Hutchinson's freckle.

Solar Keratosis

Solar keratosis (also called actinic keratosis) is a premalignant lesion caused by the additive effect of long-term sun exposure on the skin. The lesions first appear as flesh-colored to pink scaling patches located on the face, ears, arms and hands. Actinic keratoses are most common in middle-aged and elderly fair-skinned persons. The lesions feel rough to the touch, almost like sandpaper. Unless traumatized or advanced in nature, the lesions are asymptomatic.

Actinic keratoses often appear in multiples, and because they run a risk of turning cancerous, treatment is generally advised. The most common treatment is application of liquid nitrogen, which causes transient stinging. Topical creams containing the compound fluorouracil can be used to treat larger body surfaces, including the face and arm. Fluorouracil is generally applied daily over a two- to four-week period. During this time, marked redness can be anticipated. Additional topical therapies, all FDA approved for this indication, are diclofenac (Solaraze), imiquimod (Aldara) and tirbanibulin (Klisyri). Photodynamic therapy requires a special light source to activate a topically applied agent. This too is useful to treat multiple lesions. Any sites that persist despite therapy are best removed surgically and sent for biopsy to rule out carcinoma. Regular use of sunscreens will reduce the formation of keratoses in predisposed individuals. Some evidence suggests that oral nicotinamide (also called vitamin B3) may reduce the rate of pre–skin cancers in individuals at high risk.

Leukoplakia

This condition occurs as discrete white patches that arise on mucous membranes. Areas include the inside of the mouth, lips, and genitalia. Any thickened, whitish patches at these sites should be medically evaluated. Oral leukoplakia is more common in smokers.

Hutchinson's Freckle (Lentigo Maligna)

This condition occurs most frequently on the cheeks and foreheads of the elderly. It consists of a tan patch that slowly enlarges and darkens. After many years, cancer may develop, and for this reason Hutchinson's freckles should be closely monitored for changes that may indicate progression to melanoma.

SKIN CANCER

Cancer of the skin is the most common form of malignancy. Virtually all skin cancers are curable if detected and treated early. Periodic skin examinations are especially important for persons with a personal or family history of skin cancer, those middle-aged and older, and those who have experienced excessive sun exposure or tan indoors. Any suspicious changes should be brought to the attention of a medical provider trained in skin cancer recognition.

Three main types of skin cancer are recognized: basal cell carcinoma, squamous cell carcinoma, and malignant melanoma.

Basal Cell Carcinoma

Basal cell carcinoma is the most common form of cancer and accounts for nearly 70 percent of all skin cancers. This year, well over one million new cases will be diagnosed. Some 99 percent of these cancers occur in Caucasians, especially those with fair skin that burns easily. This tumor usually begins as a small, flesh-colored pimple that slowly enlarges, developing a depressed center surrounded by a smooth, shiny border. Although basal cell carcinoma rarely spreads to organs inside the body, it gradually eats away at the skin and will damage deeper tissues if left untreated. To prevent such destructive effects, tumors are best removed early in their course.

Squamous Cell Carcinoma

This cancer usually arises in skin damaged by many years of sunlight—that is, in skin excessively wrinkled, thinned, and discolored. Sun-exposed areas, such as the face, lower lip, neck, and top surface of the hands, are the most common sites. Solar (actinic) keratoses and leukoplakia (white lip patches) may turn into squamous cell carcinoma.

Squamous cell carcinoma frequently occurs as a crusted sore that fails to heal. This malignancy can spread internally to surrounding lymph nodes. Treatment usually entails surgical removal or radiation therapy. Early lesions may resolve with liquid nitrogen cryosurgery or following topical application of imiquimod or fluorouracil creams.

Malignant Melanoma

Although malignant melanoma accounts for only 3 percent of all skin cancers, it results in 65 percent of the deaths from skin cancer. In other words, malignant melanoma is an uncommon but deadly form of skin cancer. According to the American Academy of Dermatology, one American dies from skin cancer every sixty-two minutes. And the incidence of melanoma has increased significantly over the past twenty years. According to the Centers for Disease Control, the majority of melanomas are directly tied to ultraviolet light. Hereditary predisposition plays a role as well. Individuals at highest risk include those with a personal or family history of melanoma, a history of sunburn as a child, skin that easily freckles and burns, blue or green eye color, blond or red hair, and a large number of moles.

Malignant melanoma may arise on normal skin or from a preexisting birthmark or mole. This skin cancer can afflict people of all age groups, so anyone with a suspicious new growth or a change in color, size, or contour of an existing mole or birthmark should be evaluated as soon as possible. Left unchecked, melanoma can spread to the brain, lung, and lymph nodes with fatal results; detected early, the cure rate is very high.

Everyone should be aware of the ABCDEs of melanoma recognition:

Asymmetry: One side of a mole does not look like the other side.

Border: Irregular or notched borders are a danger sign.

Color: Shades of red, white, or blue are patriotic but may also signify skin cancer.

Diameter: As a general rule, moles that are smaller than a pencil eraser are OK.

Elevation or Evolving: Increased height of an existing mole warrants evaluation, as does *any* change.

And keep in mind the *ugly duckling sign* as well. Moles on a given individual tend to look alike. The ugly duckling—the one that looks different from others—is more likely to be a melanoma, even if it doesn't exhibit the classic ABCDE features.

Individuals at risk for melanoma should be examined on a regular basis. Periodic self-exams are prudent as well. Examine your body in front of a mirror, and use a hand mirror to view your neck, scalp, back, and buttocks. The key to melanoma survival is early recognition

11

Hair, Scalp, and Nails

NORMAL HAIR

THE SCALP CONTAINS APPROXIMATELY ONE HUNDRED THOUSAND HAIRS. Each hair attains a maximum length and then enters a resting stage, following which it falls out. Unlike certain animals that shed entire outer layers at once, humans have hairs that act independently; normal human hair loss occurs in random fashion and is quite inconspicuous. Some one hundred scalp hairs are regularly shed on a daily basis. This may seem like a large number, but it represents only one-thousandth of the total scalp hair.

Hair grows at different rates depending on location. Scalp hair expands at a rate of one-hundredth of an inch per day; in other words, one hundred feet of new hair is manufactured on a daily basis. Each scalp hair can grow for three to ten years. This contrasts to the hair of the armpits and eyebrows, which has a growth period of less than one year; these hairs grow to fixed lengths and enter into a prolonged resting period.

The hair that we look at, fondle, and spend so much time and money on is dead tissue. Living hair is produced from protein under the skin, within a structure called the hair follicle. The hair is no longer alive by the time it reaches the surface.

Each follicle is attached to an oil gland and is surrounded by nerves and muscles. Muscles on the extremities are sensitive to cold and contract on stimulation, pulling the hair follicle and altering the skin surface. This action gives rise to the tiny raised pimples known as goose bumps.

55

Hair differs in both amount and consistency among the various races. Whites are the hairiest, followed by blacks, with Asians being the least hirsute. Asians have the straightest hair, while blacks have the curliest.

Hair color depends on the number of pigment cells (melanin) within the hair shaft. Blond hair contains few pigment cells, and the snow-white hair of the elderly has virtually none. Red hair is due to an iron-bearing pigment.

GRAY HAIR

As we age, so does our hair. Aged hair is often whiter than gray. Many people first note loss of natural hair color in their thirties, and progression may be enhanced by stress. In women, gray hair develops on the fringes of the scalp and moves toward the crown. In men, graying begins on the sideburns, and the posterior scalp is the last area affected. To date, despite advertising claims touting over-the-counter melatonin, copper blockers, and vitamins, the only effective treatment is hair dye. Some of the aged follicles from which hair grows still contain miniscule amounts of pigment cells, and certain medications may uncommonly induce repigmentation, giving hope that the graying process may be reversible.

On occasion, hair dye can trigger an allergic reaction, hence the warning on package inserts to test the skin prior to each application. Allergic reactions appear to be on the rise as more, and younger, individuals dye their hair. The main culprit is an ingredient called paraphenylenediamine (PPD). An allergy to hair dye may result in an itchy red rash of the scalp, ears, and face, at times accompanied by swelling. Since PPD and other chemicals can be absorbed through the skin, there is concern about long-term consequences of exposure, including the potential to cause cancer.

DAMAGED HAIR: SPLIT ENDS

Since the hair visible to us is dead, and since it is constantly growing from under the scalp, any damage that occurs to hair above the skin is temporary.

Hair problems caused by the environment and improper treatment will improve, given time and correct management.

Our hair suffers from an incredible amount of physical and chemical abuse. The longer the hair, the greater the duration of this trauma. Persons with hair two feet long have ends nearly three years old. Over this period, imagine the amount of brushing, combing, pulling, curling, setting, shampooing, hot-air drying and sun, salt, and chlorinated-water exposure hair has been subjected to. Small wonder some of us have split ends.

Split ends (the frizzies) are the result of excessive trauma to hair. The condition is usually most prominent in longer hair. In moderation, combing, brushing, and blow-drying do not damage hair. When such activities are too frequently and vigorously undertaken, split ends are the inevitable result. Blow-drying is safe if it does not continue after the hair is dry to the touch. Similarly, chemical treatments, such as bleaching, waving or curling, and straightening, may also contribute to split ends.

Damage to hair can be lessened by use of conditioners and cream rinses. These compounds coat the hair surface and reduce combing friction. They also help guard against injurious effects on hair from blow-drying and sun exposure. Once they're apparent, the only cure for split ends is to cut them off.

HAIR LOSS: PATTERN ALOPECIA

As noted, an insignificant amount of hair is lost from the scalp daily. When hair is shed at a more rapid rate, the loss becomes noticeable. Such hair loss may be either generalized or confined to distinct areas.

Male pattern baldness is a hereditary disorder that first becomes apparent in late adolescence or early adulthood. Progressive hair loss is noted in the front and center of the scalp and is due to the slow shrinkage and subsequent death of hair follicles.

To date, only two products are FDA approved to slow down or reverse male pattern alopecia: topical minoxidil (Rogaine) and oral finasteride

(Propecia). A third, oral dutasteride (Avodart) is considered safe and effective but lacks FDA approval for this indication.

Minoxidil (in pill form) was first marketed as an oral treatment for high blood pressure. Problems soon became evident when the drug was administered to women and children: they began to sprout beards and mustaches.

With this in mind, clinicians began rubbing the stuff on the shiny scalps of bald men, and lo and behold, new hairs began to sprout. This was indeed a monumental accomplishment, the first time in history that something grew new hairs. Minoxidil dilates blood vessels, but the mechanism of action on scalp hairs is still unclear.

Topical minoxidil does not work on everyone. People with the least amount of hair loss and those balding for the shortest period appear to do best. For many of these individuals, minoxidil results in significant hair growth. By starting minoxidil treatment early, one may place male pattern baldness on hold. The compound is available in solution and mousse forms. Some individuals cannot tolerate daily application, due to burning and irritation.

Low-dose oral minoxidil is gaining traction as a treatment for hair loss, and several studies document both safety and efficacy in woman and men. Dosing ranges from half a milligram to five milligrams daily, much lower than the dose used to treat high blood pressure. Oral minoxidil is only available by prescription and is inexpensive. Side effects are uncommon but include lightheadedness, low blood pressure, ankle swelling, and unwanted facial hair growth.

Finasteride is used in higher doses to treat men with enlarged prostates. This oral medication (Propecia) was approved in 1997 as a treatment for male pattern baldness. The drug inhibits the breakdown of the male hormone testosterone. Finasteride can induce new hair growth in about 50 percent of men and can also increase the weight and diameter of existing hair. As is the case with minoxidil, therapy with finasteride is for life; once it's discontinued, the natural process of hair loss will proceed. Finasteride's long-term effect on general health is unknown; however, data indicates that prolonged use may actually decrease the risk of prostate cancer, a significant finding. Dutasteride (Avodart) acts in a similar manner to finasteride but has a longer half-life. In other words, daily use may not be required. On another positive note, a study published in 2009 concluded that Avodart lowered the risk of prostate cancer by 23 percent.

For those unaided by or deciding against use of either minoxidil or oral agents, depleted hair may be covered up by a toupee or hair weave or improved by hair transplantation.

Hair transplantation involves transfer of hair from the back of the scalp to depleted or thinned areas on the front and sides. In a procedure called follicular unit transplantation, thin strips of hair are removed from the posterior scalp. These are dissected into thousands of micrografts prior to transplantation. An alternative procedure involves shaving of the posterior scalp and removal of individual follicles. Tiny slits allow placement of prepared grafts beneath the skin's surface.

Certain lasers and light sources may stimulate new hair growth. Indeed, units are now available for home use. Until adequate clinical studies are published, laser and light use for baldness should be viewed with a healthy degree of skepticism.

Classic female pattern hair loss is also called androgenetic alopecia. The condition most commonly occurs around menopause and characteristically involves the front and top of the scalp. Treatment with minoxidil may stabilize the condition. Rogaine for women is available in a 5 percent concentration, which is superior to the 2 percent formulation. To avoid unwanted facial hair, users should take care to apply minoxidil only to the scalp and let it thoroughly dry before resting the head on a pillow. Minoxidil should not be used by pregnant or nursing females. As mentioned, low-dose oral minoxidil is gaining in popularity as a treatment for hair thinning and loss. The main side effect is unwanted hair growth elsewhere, such as on the face and arms.

More uncommon adverse reactions include ankle swelling and headaches. Be patient; maximal results may take up to six months.

The oral medication spironolactone helps to block male hormone uptake by the hair follicle, although clinical response is slow. Spironolactone will not improve hair loss due to nonhormonal factors, such as stress and chemotherapy. One study found that the majority of women with female pattern hair loss on this medication noticed improvement, and another study demonstrated that the combination of spironolactone with topical minoxidil led to decreased hair shedding and increased hair growth.

Minigraft hair transplantation is another option for women and may yield excellent cosmetic results. Use of finasteride and dutasteride in postmenopausal women with hair loss is advocated by some dermatologists. Platelet-rich plasma (PRP) is an alternative treatment for androgenetic alopecia in both males and females. This process involves drawing blood, which is then processed and injected into the scalp. Multiple sessions are required, and results vary.

Want fuller eyelashes? In 2008, the prescription eyelash-enhancer Latisse (bimatoprost) became available. Applied like eyeliner, Latisse enters eyelash hair follicles and results in longer, thicker, and darker eyelashes. It's not cheap, but it works.

HAIR LOSS: TELOGEN EFFLUVIUM

Generalized hair loss in women can result from a variety of stressful situations. For example, increased hair shedding frequently follows pregnancy. The loss of hair ranges from mild to extensive and may manifest from the first to twelfth week after delivery. No treatment is necessary, as the hair completely grows back. Such hair loss is referred to as *telogen effluvium*.

Women taking birth control pills may experience diffuse hair thinning, either while on these pills or shortly following their discontinuation. Again, this hair loss is only temporary and fully corrects itself within a few months.

Serious infections can also lead to temporary hair loss, and many cases are attributed to COVID.

HAIR LOSS: ALOPECIA AREATA

Alopecia areata is a common form of localized hair loss that affects both children and adults. The condition usually presents as a circular zone of complete hair loss, revealing portions of the scalp that are smooth and shiny. Involved sites may range from dime-sized to larger than a silver dollar. A small percentage of alopecia areata patients will progress to total loss of scalp hair (alopecia totalis) or even lose eyebrow, armpit, and groin hairs (alopecia universalis). The cosmetic and psychological effects can be devastating.

Alopecia areata results from an abnormal immune response directed against hair follicles. Some cases follow emotional stress and tension. Fortunately, most of the hairless patches spontaneously sprout hair in several months. Dermatologists treat localized forms of this disorder with topical steroids or steroid injections. In 2022, Olumiant (baricitinib, a so-called JAK inhibitor) was approved by the FDA to treat severe alopecia areata, and in 2023, a second JAK inhibitor, Litfulo (ritlecitinib) was approved as well. Both are pills taken by mouth. Results are variable, but many patients experience significant hair growth. The National Alopecia Areata Foundation is an excellent resource for those seeking additional information (naaf.org).

HAIR LOSS: TRAUMATIC

Some anxious individuals consciously or subconsciously pull at and twist their hair until breakage occurs. This compulsive behavior is called trichotillomania and results in patchy zones of hair loss, within which broken hairs of uneven length are found. Chronic cases warrant psychiatric consultation.

Various cosmetic manipulations can lead to hair loss. Traction produced by tight rollers or braids may weaken the hair as it exits the scalp, leading to patchy areas of thinning or even baldness. The kinky hair of blacks is particularly prone to fracture. Such traction alopecia is usually most noticeable on the sides of the scalp.

Bleaching, setting, and permanent wave solutions will not significantly damage hair unless applied in an inappropriately high concentration or over a prolonged time. However, the frequent use of hot combs and oils to straighten hair (a cultural adaptation practiced by many African Americans) may cause marked scarring of the scalp and permanent baldness. Hot-comb alopecia most commonly occurs in the center of the scalp.

Several hair myths are just that. The plucking of hair does not produce permanent baldness (nor does it cause hair to grow thicker). Cutting, shaving, or massaging the scalp has no effect on hair growth. Frequent hair washing and shampooing also do not lead to hair loss, nor does dandruff (no matter how severe).

A WORD ABOUT HAIR PRODUCTS

In 2023, the FDA proposed a rule banning formaldehyde and other formaldehyde-releasing chemicals from being used in hair-smoothing and straightening products, due to long-term health concerns. A study published in 2019 linked hair dye and chemical straightener use to an increased risk of breast cancer in women. Further, a 2022 study found that women who used hair-straightening chemicals had an increased risk of developing uterine cancer. Black women are disproportionately at higher risk.

EXCESS HAIR

Excess hair growth is termed *hirsutism*. For most, the problem is simply a cosmetic one and not indicative of the presence of hormonal or gender abnormalities. If one examined a group of white females, nearly one-quarter would be found to have hair on the upper lip (with the condition being very apparent in 10 percent), and more than three-quarters would exhibit coarse hair on their arms and legs.

Hair distribution is in large part genetically determined; if your mother has excess facial hair, you most likely will too. In general, women of southern Mediterranean and Near Eastern origin have more facial and body hair than do North American and Asian women.

About 1 percent of women complaining of excess body hair have a significant medical problem, such as overactive adrenal glands or ovaries. These women may also experience menstrual irregularities, weight gain, and acne. Some drugs, such as Depo-Provera, Dilantin, and tamoxifen, can also induce hirsutism.

Several modalities are used to remove unwanted hairs, with the current gold standard being lasers and intense pulsed light (IPL).

Lasers and IPL are specialized light sources. Light used for hair removal passes through the skin and is absorbed by pigment within the hair follicle. The procedure can be safely performed on virtually any part of the body, except about the eyes. Hair that is coarse and dark responds best to laser treatment. Blond, white, or red hair is difficult to treat. As the pulses of light energy are of brief duration, discomfort is momentary.

Laser and IPL hair removal usually requires multiple sessions. Approximately 20 to 30 percent reduction will be noted after each treatment, with long-term hair reduction approaching 90 percent. Treatments are repeated every four to six weeks, depending on location (shorter time intervals are required for hairs above the neck). Note that the FDA allows approved manufacturers to claim "permanent reduction" but not "permanent removal" for their devices.

Side effects associated with laser and IPL hair removal are transient redness, inflammation of the hair follicles (folliculitis), activation of fever blisters, pigmentary changes, and (rarely) scarring.

Light-based hair-reduction devices for home use are available. These appear to be safe and somewhat effective. Make sure that any light or laser device marketed for hair reduction is approved by the FDA before purchase, but note that FDA approval does not equate to efficacy.

Unsightly hair may be removed by electrolysis. In this procedure, a tiny needle is placed within each hair follicle, and a short burst of current is administered. The electrical charge destroys the follicle and prevents further hair growth. Electrolysis is the only hair-removal modality the FDA calls permanent. The procedure is time-consuming and somewhat painful. Results range from acceptable to excellent. Electrolysis is a viable alternative to treat light blond, white, and gray hairs, as these respond poorly to light-based treatments.

Shaving with either a safety razor or an electric shaver is a simple, temporary means of hair removal. As noted, repeated shaving or plucking with tweezers does not lead to increased or thickened hair growth. Hair plucking pulls the hair from the root. Results last about six weeks.

Depilatory creams are another means of hair removal. These compounds cause a transient dissolution of surface hair following a brief application time ranging from five to ten minutes. Their use on sensitive skin may cause irritation.

Objectionable hairs may be rendered inconspicuous through bleaching. Again, this is a simple, albeit temporary, measure to improve the cosmetic impact of excess facial hair.

DANDRUFF: SEBORRHEIC DERMATITIS

The medical term for dandruff is *seborrheic dermatitis*. This condition tends to affect hair-bearing regions and facial furrows. It is a disorder not of hair but of the underlying skin. *Seborrhea* literally means "freely flowing sebum," and the problem occurs in areas with a large number of oil glands. Common sites include the scalp, eyebrows, central face, external ear, midchest, upper back, belly button, and genital areas.

The most common form of seborrheic dermatitis is that of greasy, scaling dandruff, the white flecks that stand out on dark-colored clothing. Severe seborrheic dermatitis manifests as inflamed, scaling bright red patches located on the scalp, face, and chest, which may also spread to armpits and the groin.

Mild cases of seborrhea are managed with over-the-counter remedies. Active ingredients in dandruff shampoos include selenium sulfide (Head & Shoulders, Selsun Blue), zinc pyrithione (DHS Zinc), tar (DHS Tar, Neutrogena T/Gel, Tarsum), and ketoconazole (Nizoral), which also are available in a cream formulation. One percent hydrocortisone cream or lotion helps minimize redness and scaling. Stubborn cases may require prescription topical steroids.

To be effective, a dandruff shampoo should remain on the scalp for at least five to ten minutes before rinsing. Over time, a shampoo may lose effectiveness. Should this occur, the best course of action is to switch to another type of shampoo. Those with a more severe form of seborrhea may require cortisone in the form of a gel, foam, spray, or lotion prescribed by a physician. Seborrheic dermatitis affecting the face (characterized by redness and scaling of the forehead and skin folds) may respond to low-potency topical steroids, antifungals (such as ketoconazole), or pimecrolimus (Elidel). In 2023, Zoryve foam (roflumilast) became the first topical drug approved by the FDA to treat seborrheic dermatitis.

NAILS

Our nails are made of keratin, a rock-hard, shiny substance. Analogous to hair, the nail itself is dead. The living part of the nail lies under the skin, in a region called the matrix, and it is here that new keratin is formed. Any physical damage inflicted on the outer nail is temporary, as new keratin is constantly being produced by the matrix. Fingernails grow at a rate of one-eighth of an inch per month, and toenails grow even slower. If a fingernail is lost, about six months are required for a new one to completely grow back. Regrowth of a toenail might take more than a year. By contrast, damage to the matrix may lead to gross distortion and permanent loss of the affected nail.

Deformities of the nail may be caused by trauma, fungal infections, and diseases, such as psoriasis. Nail discoloration is often due to physical factors; for example, a black nail results from injury, and a yellow nail results from cigarette smoking. Greenish nails are caused by a pigment-secreting bacterium called *Pseudomonas*. The tiny white flecks that adorn many nails are usually induced by minor insults, such as excess nail filing or nail biting. Sometimes nail changes indicate serious internal disease. Clubbed nails may be a sign of lung cancer; spoon-shaped nails may be a sign of anemia. The bed of the fingernails should be light pink. White nail beds are a sign of anemia. Nails that are white and opaque may be a sign of liver disease, whereas half-and-half nails (bottom white and top pink) may indicate kidney disease. Although a black nail is usually the result of trauma, be careful; pigment under a nail may represent melanoma, a serious form of skin cancer.

Nails, like hair, are made of protein. Nail strength and texture may be adversely affected by nutritional deficiencies, but in a healthy person, strength and enhanced texture will not be improved by the ingestion of excess protein or calcium. The notion that gelatin enhances nail growth and luster is simply a myth.

Many women complain of brittle nails. This distressing but harmless condition is caused by microscopic loss of water from keratin. Soaking nails in lukewarm water and then applying a moisturizing ointment may prove of benefit. Data supporting the use of the B vitamin biotin as a treatment for brittle nails is inconclusive. Further, in 2017, the FDA issued a statement warning the public of the harmful effects of high-dose biotin on laboratory testing. The FDA concluded that biotin supplements pose a risk to public safety.

Fingernail length is a matter of personal preference. Because toenails are subjected to weight bearing and close confinement, their length should be curtailed by proper trimming. Each toenail is best squared off when cut, not clipped too deeply, which allows the sides of the nail to contact skin. Improper cutting of toenails, as well as ill-fitting footwear and improper gait, leads to ingrown toenails, a troublesome condition that may warrant surgical correction.

Applying polish to nails is a safe procedure that has no effect on nail health and growth. Very rarely, a woman may develop an allergy to nail polish, characterized by redness and itching wherever the substance contacts skin. A greater risk of allergy is from compounds used in nail sculpturing, and many have been taken off the market for this reason. Acrylic nails cause little harm, unless left on for too long. Best practice is to remove them at least once every three months and to allow two to three weeks prior to reapplication.

Swelling at the base of a nail is called paronychia; the affected area is red and tender. Paronychias of long-standing duration are seen almost exclusively in women. Underlying causes are yeast infection and chronic environmental stress, which includes repeated contact with detergents and solvents. Keeping the nail as dry as possible is an important component of therapy. Improvement may follow application of a topical steroid or antiyeast cream.

One of the most common nail problems is caused by fungi. Fungal infection of the nail begins at the free margins and sides and results in yellowish discoloration, increased thickness, and marked fragility. Toenails are more frequently affected than fingernails.

Nail fungal infections are often embarrassing due to distortion and color changes. Oral therapy offers the best chance of cure or extended remission. Terbinafine (Lamisil) is considered the drug of choice and remains affordable, with a good safety record. FDA-approved antifungal topical solutions are Jublia (efinaconazole), Kerydin (tavaborole), and

Stephen M. Schleicher, MD

Penlac (ciclopirox). These should be applied to affected nails daily and must be continued for months to be effective. Lasers are currently in vogue and heavily advertised. Therapy is expensive, and the results are questionable. Surgical removal of an infected nail is another option.

Psoriasis can affect nails, leading to pitting, yellow-brown discoloration, and increased thickness. Over time, nails may loosen and separate from the nail bed. The condition may be painful and associated with arthritis. The most effective treatment is with biologics (discussed in an upcoming chapter).

12

Cellulite and Stretch Marks

CELLULITE IS A COSMETIC NUISANCE OF AESTHETIC CONCERN TO millions of women. Indeed, the condition affects more than 80 percent of postpubertal females. Cellulite treatment is now a multimillion-dollar industry ranging from over-the-counter creams to injectable dissolvents, mechanical devices, and lasers.

Cellulite is not a disease but the result of a naturally occurring process that affects the thighs and buttocks of women as they age. Over time, the fat cells in these areas become less organized and lax, giving rise to the lumps and depressions that characterize this condition. Factors that contribute to the severity of cellulite are heredity and obesity. If your mother has significant cellulite, chances are good that you will too. The risk of cellulite increases if one is overweight and out of shape. Cellulite is not associated with physical discomfort. Men are not affected, because of the lesser amount of fat (adipose tissue) in locations where cellulite typically forms.

Individuals with cellulite may benefit from weight reduction and a muscle-toning exercise routine. Crash dieting is to be avoided, as drastic loss of weight may worsen the appearance. Some report improvement with daily massage, stroking the skin with the hand or a brush. Topical creams containing caffeine or retinol are claimed to benefit milder cases, although any improvement is usually short-lived.

Several physical modalities are used to treat cellulite. One, termed *extracorporeal shock wave therapy*, employs electrical energy to disrupt underlying tissue. This results in collagen remodeling and improves localized circulation. Similar results may be achieved with both acoustic (sound) wave therapy and radiofrequency devices. Multiple sessions are required.

Laser- and light-based devices are also used to treat cellulite. These work by stimulating fibroblasts and collagen. Results are usually modest. Enhanced results have been reported with a subdermal laser technique that leads to heat damage to fat cells and dissolution of fibrous bands. Another minimally invasive procedure is tissue stabilized-guided subcision: under local anesthesia, fibrous bands responsible for dimpling are cleaved.

Improvement of cellulite has been reported with injection of the collagen-dissolving enzyme *Clostridium histolyticum*. The injection takes about fifteen minutes and is administered in three-week intervals. Results can last up to two years. Improvement has also been achieved with injections of diluted calcium hydroxylapatite and poly-l-lactic acid microspheres. These agents increase collagen and elastin. As with all treatment modalities, studies are ongoing to assess longevity. Therapies are safe, although temporary bruising is to be expected.

Stretch marks, medically termed *striae distensae*, are a form of scar tissue that affects the dermal layer. They initially appear as pink, reddened, or purplish lesions that whiten over time. Affected areas include the breasts, abdomen, hips, thighs, buttocks, and upper arms.

Stretch marks are most commonly associated with pregnancy, developing to some degree in approximately 75 percent of women prior to delivery. Contributing factors include weight gain and hormonal changes. Stretch marks can also occur in men, especially those who rapidly gain muscle mass as a consequence of weightlifting with or without illicit steroids.

Prevention is difficult. Avoidance of rapid weight gain or loss is advised. Steroids taken to gain muscle mass are potentially dangerous and may induce not only striae but also more serious medical conditions. Pregnant women may benefit from a combination of moisturizers and massage.

Treatment of stretch marks is best undertaken at an early stage when the lesions are discolored. One goal of therapy is to hasten the conversion of reddened or purplish patches to lighter, less visible hues, and hydrocortisone cream is worth a trial. Topical retinoids, such as Aklief, Differin, and Retin-A, promote production of collagen and can improve stretch marks. Several studies document improvement following laser, IPL, and fractional photothermolysis. These therapies reduce the redness associated with striae and may increase skin elasticity. Multiple treatment sessions are usually required.

13

Dilated Blood Vessels

TELANGIECTASIAS

Minute dilated blood vessels (enlarged capillaries) are medically termed *telangiectasias*. They appear as thin red strands (called *spiders*) that lose their color upon application of pressure. Since the vessels are permanently dilated, the color promptly returns when the pressure is removed.

Most telangiectasias are found on the face, but they may also occur on the chest and back. Spiders are frequently encountered and are most prominent in fair-skinned individuals. They increase in number with age and with excessive sun exposure. Pregnant women may develop multiple telangiectasias, as may persons suffering from chronic alcoholism and liver disease. One of the hallmarks of rosacea is the appearance of facial telangiectasias.

Spiders are harmless, but they are often a cosmetic nuisance. Electrocautery using a tiny needle will eradicate solitary lesions. Multiple lesions are best treated with light devices, including pulsed dye laser (PDL) and intense pulsed light (IPL). Temporary bruising is the only adverse consequence.

CHERRY ANGIOMAS

Cherry angiomas are bright red dots that appear on the skin surface and are commonly found in individuals after the age of forty. The most common location is the trunk. Cherry angiomas are composed of thin blood vessels, which first appear as pinpoint dots and gradually enlarge, at times reaching the size of a pencil eraser. They are painless and harmless but cosmetically unappealing. If they're traumatized, profuse bleeding will result. The lesions can be removed simply by either electrocautery or a laser.

LEG VEINS

As a person ages, blood vessels (venules) within the calves and thighs expand in diameter. Varicose veins are larger vessels that range in color from flesh-toned to dark blue and often have a bulging, cord-like appearance. Spider veins are smaller in size and closer to the surface. Often, they network in a pattern similar to a tree branch. Hereditary predisposition, obesity, prolonged standing, hormonal changes, and pregnancy are contributory factors, and more than 50 percent of women are affected.

Spider veins have no medical significance but are unsightly. The most common treatment is sclerotherapy; this entails injection of the offending vessels with a sclerosing agent administered through a tiny needle. The procedure is accomplished without local anesthesia, and discomfort is usually momentary and minimal. When sclerotherapy is performed by an experienced health-care provider, complications are infrequent and not serious; at times, bruising occurs, but this gradually fades. Skin breakdown (ulceration) may result if injected material leaks into surrounding tissue. Common sclerosing agents include sodium tetradecyl sulfate, polidocanol, and hypertonic saline (concentrated salt solution). Following injection, a compression bandage should be applied for twenty-four hours. A successful injection produces dissolution of the dilated vessel over a three- to six-week period.

Laser therapy is a more costly solution and works best on the vessels of tiniest diameter. Minute bursts of intense light are directed into the veins, and fading gradually ensues. Although somewhat painful, laser treatment avoids needles and may be the only option when blood vessels are too narrow for injection. Often, two to five treatments are required for adequate cosmetic result. As with sclerotherapy, there is no downtime.

Varicose veins can be a sign of venous insufficiency. At times, they may ache. Workup entails physical examination and, on occasion, ultrasound analysis.

Sclerotherapy is often an option. Larger vessels may be surgically removed by phlebectomy or stripping with ligation. These procedures are best performed in a surgicenter or hospital and entail small excisions followed by dissection of the offending vessels.

A newer therapy called endovenous ablation entails the insertion of a catheter that emits radiofrequency energy into the vein. Alternatively, laser light can be administered using a fiber. The end result is shrinkage of the vein wall.

Bear in mind that a key to the prevention or recurrence of leg veins is compression. For predisposed individuals, graduated-support compression stockings are recommended for use during daytime hours.

BRUISING: SENILE PURPURA

Bruising in the elderly is not uncommon and merits its own name: *senile purpura* (*purpura* is the medical term for bruising). The condition manifests as irregularly shaped dark purple blotches that arise primarily on the arms and back of the hands.

Aged skin loses connective tissue, and blood vessels become more fragile. These circumstances are worsened by chronic exposure to sunlight. In predisposed individuals, even the slightest trauma can rupture superficial capillaries and veins, resulting in bruising.

Senile purpura is cosmetically unappealing but, fortunately, not a sign of an underlying disease or vitamin deficiency. Affected areas are not painful and do not itch. Lesions gradually fade over two to three weeks but may leave behind a persistent yellowish-to-brown discoloration. Several creams are marketed to improve the appearance of bruised skin, and many contain extracts of the herb arnica. Whether these hasten the healing process is open to conjecture.

14

Perspiration

HUMANS PERSPIRE, AND EACH YEAR, AMERICAN CONSUMERS SPEND some $750 million on underarm products designed to inhibit sweating and prevent offensive odor. Perspiration occurs throughout the body, but it is most abundant in the underarm and genital areas, owing to the large accumulation of sweat glands at these sites. Newly formed sweat is acted on by bacteria to produce the characteristic body odor, known to every kid as BO. A deodorant either masks this odor or decreases its production by inhibiting some of the underarm bacteria. Antiperspirants, on the other hand, act by reducing the flow of glandular perspiration. Commonly used antiperspirants frequently contain aluminum compounds that inhibit sweat production.

Antiperspirants and deodorants are marketed in a variety of forms, including creams, roll-ons, and aerosols. The first two are more efficient and cost-effective; the latter is more convenient. With the increasing concern over personal health and the environment, the use of aerosols has been curtailed.

Antiperspirants and deodorants are generally safe and effective. If mild burning or irritation develops, switch to another brand. Baking soda (sodium bicarbonate) works well, and those with sensitive skin might consider using this inexpensive, readily available compound.

EXCESSIVE PERSPIRATION: HYPERHIDROSIS

It is, of course, normal to sweat, but some are plagued by an exaggerated sweat response. Called hyperhidrosis, this distressing condition may affect the palms and soles as well as the underarms, face, and scalp. Profuse sweating is triggered by heat, physical activity, or stress. The hands, feet, and underarms produce a steady stream of moisture ("sweating buckets"), leading to marked self-consciousness in most hyperhidrosis sufferers. Survey data suggests that more than one million Americans are negatively impacted by excess sweating.

Hyperhidrosis often begins during puberty and improves with age. Topical therapy with a nonprescription clinical-strength or extrastrength antiperspirant should be the first line of therapy. Examples include Certain Dri, Secret Clinical Strength, Dove Invisible Solid, and Degree Invisible Solid. The ideal time for application is at bedtime, as these agents work best when applied to dry skin. A deodorant may be applied in the morning for cosmetic purpose. Persons not achieving adequate control may benefit from prescription topical antiperspirants Drysol or Qbrexza. The active ingredient of Drysol is 20 percent aluminum chloride. Qbrexza contains glycopyrronium, which has been used in pill form for years to prevent excess sweating, under the tradename Robinul. Another oral medication used for this purpose is Ditropan (oxybutynin). Higher doses of either product may lead to dry mouth.

Iontophoresis (Drionic) therapy uses a battery-powered device to inhibit excess sweating of the hands, feet, and underarms. The small current induces electrical charges in the sweat glands that decrease sweat production. The treatment is safe, but relief is variable, and therapy must be continued indefinitely. The MiraDry system is a microwave energy device used to treat underarm hyperhidrosis by selective heating of the sweat glands. Treatment results in irreversible loss of these glands. Cost is significant, and side effects are common, including localized post-treatment swelling, redness, and discomfort. Many patients express satisfaction with the end result.

The botulinum neurotoxins Botox, Dysport, and Xeomin, when injected into the underarms, palms, and soles (and even into the face and scalp), are effective modalities commonly used to minimize hyperhidrosis and are considered the gold standard of therapy. Drawbacks include transient discomfort during injection (multiple sticks are required) as well as high cost, which may not be covered by insurance. Injections need to be repeated every six to nine months. The majority of individuals treated with botulinum neurotoxins achieve satisfaction with this procedure. In 2023, the FDA approved a physician-applied patch (Brella) to combat underarm sweating. When it's applied for three minutes, results are said to last two to four months.

Surgical excision or liposuction may be used to remove sweat glands situated within the armpits. A more drastic option is surgical destruction of the nerves that control sweat production (sympathectomy), a procedure generally reserved for incapacitating sweating.

15

Acne

Do zits give you fits? Chances are, yes. Acne is the most common skin problem, affecting, to some degree, three out of every four teenagers and many in their twenties and thirties. The problem is an expensive one, with multimillions of dollars spent each year on over-the-counter preparations as well as prescription drugs. For many, acne consists of nothing more than an occasional pimple or blemish on the face, back, or chest. A few are less fortunate and develop extensive, persistent eruptions that result in permanent pits and scars. The psychological effects may be devastating, and acne has been linked to depression and suicidal thoughts.

Acne is dependent on the presence of sebaceous (oil) glands found within the dermis. These specialized structures are most numerous on the face but are also located on the back, chest, and upper arms. At puberty, the glands undergo rapid enlargement due to hormonal stimulation. As the glands grow in size, they become more active, manufacturing a mixture of oils that, in excessive amounts, gives rise to the so-called oily complexion. The gland openings (pores) may become clogged, causing the oil, or sebum, to back up and stagnate. Bacteria growing in the sebum break down this substance into a number of irritating compounds that lead to the formation of blackheads, whiteheads, and those unsightly mountains and craters affectionately called zits.

There are several different types of acne lesions. These include comedones (whiteheads and blackheads), papules, pustules, cysts, and scars. Comedones are of two varieties: open and closed. A closed comedone, called a whitehead, arises from a pore clogged with oil. Sebum creates a tiny white covering over the entrance. When the opening remains unobstructed, the oil is oxidized by the air and turns black. This open type of comedone is called a blackhead.

A papule is a solid, elevated lesion of the skin. Papules range in hue from flesh-colored to bright red. Red papules are pimples undergoing inflammation.

A pustule is a pimple filled with fluid, or pus. This substance is composed of dead cells and bacteria. When a pustule becomes larger and deeper, it is then termed a *cyst*. Tender, inflamed red pustules and cysts may result in scars, which is the reason these two lesion types represent the most severe forms of acne.

What is the cause of acne? Why do some people escape this condition entirely, while others are plagued with blemishes, zits, and blackheads year after year?

Acne has been linked to a number of factors, including heredity. If one of your parents had acne, you run an increased risk of developing this condition as well.

Hormones may also play a role in the development of acne. For many, acne first becomes a problem in puberty. During this period, testosterone, the male sex hormone, is formed not only by the male sex organs but also, in small quantities, by the ovaries in young women. Testosterone causes marked growth of the sebaceous glands and, in susceptible persons, may trigger or worsen acne.

Some females develop one or two pimples each month shortly before their menstrual periods. Others may experience flare-ups when placed on certain birth control pills. In both cases, the resultant acne is due to changes in the body's hormone levels. Polycystic ovary syndrome is characterized by irregular periods, excess facial hair, and scalp hair thinning. Abnormal hormone levels in women with this disorder lead to persistent acne. Persons undergoing female-to-male transformation often develop acne due to administration of testosterone.

Many women first develop acne not at puberty or in adolescence but during their twenties and thirties. Prolonged use of cosmetics may be a factor. Moisturizers, creams, and cover-ups contribute to pore plugging and creation of comedones and papules. Some postulate that stresses of modern life subtly alter hormone levels, which in turn triggers breakouts.

A major factor that contributes to acne at any age and in either sex is the bacteria that live within the sebaceous glands. Germs break down the skin's natural oils into irritating by-products that play a key role in inflammatory lesions.

Certain factors once thought to cause and perpetuate acne are now considered unimportant. No evidence exists that lack of regular washing leads to a worsening of acne. By the same token, acne is not improved by incessant cleansing. Washing two or three times daily is all that is usually needed to remove excess oil and germs on the skin's surface.

Lingering controversy surrounds the role of diet. A diet high in fats and oils does not make the skin oilier; greasy skin is not caused by greasy foods. A years-old study was unable to demonstrate that feeding individuals with acne huge quantities of chocolate led to increased pimple formation. More recently, a link has been postulated between breakouts and high-glycemic-load diets rich in processed carbohydrates. In one study, acne severity decreased in volunteers who maintained low-carbohydrate diets.

Speaking of hormones, the role of milk in acne causation is also controversial. A recent study found a positive association between milk intake and acne. Since the majority of milk comes from pregnant cows, a tenable hypothesis holds that hormones in milk have a stimulatory effect on the oil glands of those who drink it. Another theory postulates that milk, in combination with high levels of processed refined foods and sugars, triggers acne by altering insulin levels. Skim milk appears to be the worst culprit.

For most, acne merely represents a temporary embarrassment, while for some, the condition constitutes a disfiguring disease. Regardless of the extent of involvement, virtually all cases will significantly improve with proper therapy.

Certain general principles are best followed when dealing with acne. As mentioned, it is advisable to wash the affected areas twice daily to remove excess sebum and bacteria from the skin's surface. Acne cleansers and soaps often contain surfactants that facilitate oil removal. Cleansers containing benzoyl peroxide and salicylic acid are effective. Defatting solutions known as astringents may aid in the temporary removal of surface film. Abrasive cleansers contain fine granules that are rubbed against the skin to produce a mild sandpaper effect. Such preparations will help reduce excess oil but can cause increased peeling and may prove too harsh for some people; dermatologists discourage their use in the inflammatory types of acne. Nonirritating, noncomedogenic soaps are recommended for those with sensitive skin. Pimple patches are currently in vogue and are used as spot therapy. These are a better option than picking at your zits.

Persons with acne must avoid picking, scratching, squeezing, or otherwise manipulating their pimple-plagued skin. Unless properly instructed, leave all mechanical manipulations to a skin-care specialist. The temptation is great to force out pus bumps and pop zits. But such facial trauma, besides coating the bathroom mirror, may transform an ordinary pimple into a permanent scar.

Sunlight often plays a beneficial role in acne treatment. Many experience considerable improvement during the summer months. Of course, one must weigh this benefit against any harmful long-term effects of ultraviolet radiation. Further, some acne therapies do not mix with sunlight.

Persons with acne often try over-the-counter acne preparations as first-line treatment. Active ingredients may include sulfur, resorcinol, benzoyl peroxide, salicylic acid, or alcohol. All promote drying and peeling and help limit bacterial growth.

Those who do not respond to the above measures should seek medical consultation. Dermatologists and dermatologist-trained practitioners have at their disposal a number of powerful therapeutic modalities to improve one's appearance and—of equal importance—to prevent scars.

ACNE AND TRANSGENDER MEN

More than 7 percent of American adults self-identify as lesbian, gay, bisexual, transgender, or something other than heterosexual, which is double the percentage from a decade ago. Acne may be precipitated or worsened by testosterone supplementation in trans men and may impact self-esteem, social interaction, and quality of life. Testosterone-induced acne typically occurs within the first year of commencing therapy and can affect the face, chest, and back with varying degrees of severity. Those with moderate to severe disease are urged to seek dermatological care.

ACNE THERAPIES

Benzoyl Peroxide

One of the mainstays of acne therapy is application of benzoyl peroxide. Preparations containing this substance promote facial drying and are antibacterial, leading to rapid reduction of inflammatory lesions.

Benzoyl peroxide is formulated in several concentrations, ranging from 2.5 percent to 10 percent. In general, one should start therapy with the lowest concentration. The major side effects encountered with this product are excessive dryness, irritation, and allergic reactions. As these untoward reactions increase with higher concentrations and several studies have failed to demonstrate significantly improved efficacy with higher dosing, most individuals are best maintained on lower strengths. Those with sensitive skin may not be able to tolerate this compound. Note as well that benzoyl peroxide will stain clothing.

Benzoyl peroxide is a potent oxidizing agent that kills germs on contact. Unlike antibiotics, bacteria do not develop resistance to this agent.

Over-the-counter formulations containing benzoyl peroxide include Clean and Clear, Oxy, and Proactiv. Prescription benzoyl peroxide may be combined with the topical antibiotic clindamycin (Acanya, BenzaClin, Duac, Onexton) or a topical retinoid (Epiduo, Twyneo). Cabtreo is a triple-combination acne gel that contains clindamycin, a retinoid, and benzoyl peroxide.

Sulfur

Sulfur-containing compounds have been used to treat acne since the 1800s. Sulfur has anti-inflammatory activity, and many formulations have a distinctive odor. Some sulfur-based products are available over the counter (for example, Rezamid), while others require a prescription (e.g., Avar and Klaron).

Retinoids

Topical vitamin A derivatives called retinoids are commonly used to treat acne. Examples include Aklief (trifarotene), Arazlo (tazarotene), Atralin (tretinoin), Differin (adapalene), Retin-A (tretinoin), and Tazorac (tazarotene). These substances possess comedolytic properties; they dislodge dried sebum and help keep the pores open. Retinoids may also exert a direct anti-inflammatory effect upon the follicle. The major downside of such therapy is undue irritation.

The majority of vitamin A derivatives utilized as acne therapy require a prescription; Differin gel is available over the counter. Facial redness, peeling, and burning are undesirable side effects. These reactions frequently diminish with repeated use.

Skin treated with retinoids may become very sensitive to sunlight and easily sunburned. For this reason, excess sun exposure should be minimized. In fact, at least in the summer months, prescription retinoids are best applied only at night and thoroughly washed off in the morning. Use sparingly. A pea-sized amount should be enough to cover one's entire face.

Antibiotics

The topical antibiotic clindamycin is available in solution, gel, pledget, and foam formulations (Cleocin T, Evoclin). Azelaic acid (Azelex, Finacea) is an antibacterial cream derived from wheat. Dapsone gel (Aczone) is another topical antibiotic approved as acne therapy, as is minocycline foam (Amzeeq).

As mentioned, a topical antibiotic may be combined with benzoyl peroxide therapy to decrease the potential for bacterial resistance. Clindamycin is also effective when combined with a retinoid (Ziana).

Oral antibiotics are the mainstay of therapy for moderate to severe acne. Generally, antibiotic treatment for this condition begins with a tetracycline derivative, such as doxycycline (e.g., nongeneric Acticlate and Doryx) or minocycline (e.g., Minocin and Solodyn). Oral tetracyclines have been used to treat acne for decades, and these drugs have an admirable safety record. The lowest dose of an antibiotic necessary to control acne is a prudent course of action, with discontinuation recommended once adequate control is achieved. A third-generation tetracycline, sarecycline (Seysara), may be taken with or without food and is approved to treat acne down to age nine.

Tetracycline derivatives are best not taken with milk or vitamin-mineral combinations, because these substances impede stomach absorption. They should not be administered to pregnant or nursing women or to children under the age of eight, as teeth staining may result.

Minocycline can cause dizziness (vertigo) and has been linked to blood-chemistry abnormalities and skin pigmentation. Doxycycline may uncommonly cause sun photosensitivity.

Contraceptive and Hormonal Agents

Although some oral contraceptives can worsen acne, others may reduce oil production and promote acne clearing. Women with persistent acne who do not respond to topical therapies may be candidates for such therapy.

Several birth control pills, including Ortho Tri-Cyclen (ethinyl estradiol and norgestimate), Estrostep (norethindrone-e.estradiol-iron), and Yaz (drospirenone and ethinyl estradiol), have been approved as treatment. The drug spironolactone helps counteract male hormones and is often used to treat women with moderate to severe breakouts. This relatively inexpensive drug demonstrates a high level of efficacy but may take several months to attain maximum effect.

The topical antiandrogen Winlevi (clascoterone) was approved by the FDA to treat acne in 2020. This medication decreases sebum production and can be used by both females and males.

Isotretinoin

The treatment of severe acne was revolutionized in 1982 with the approval of isotretinoin (then trade-named Accutane, now under brand names Absorica, Absorica LD, Amnesteem, Claravis, Myorisan, Sotret, Zenatane). This so-called miracle drug is a derivative of vitamin A and is available in capsule form, usually taken for five to six months. With isotretinoin, more than 80 percent of severe acne sufferers are cured of this condition. By preventing cysts and reddened papules, isotretinoin prevents the dreaded sequela of acne scarring.

Daily doses of isotretinoin range from ten to eighty milligrams, dependent in part on weight and severity. Persons on this medication experience varying degrees of dryness. Cracked lips and even nosebleeds may occur, along with temporary elevation of blood lipids. Everything normalizes once the course of isotretinoin is completed.

Controversy exists regarding the association of isotretinoin with mood changes, depression, and colitis; direct links, if they do occur, are very uncommon. Regarding the latter, trial lawyers had a field day suing manufactures for alleged causation of inflammatory bowel disease (IBD). A large population-based study published in 2014 concluded that isotretinoin did not cause this condition, and a 2022 study found that patients with IBD taking isotretinoin did not experience worsening of their condition. As for depression and suicide, studies have documented an increased risk of suicidal ideation in persons with uncontrolled acne, and one analysis found that the rate of suicide for every one hundred thousand individuals taking isotretinoin was actually lower than national rates. Indeed, the clearing effect of isotretinoin assuredly enhances the emotional well-being of those suffering from more severe forms of acne.

Isotretinoin must *never* be taken by pregnant women, because of the high probability of birth defects. Women of childbearing potential must practice strict birth control or abstinence. Persons on this drug must be registered in a central government-mandated database called iPLEDGE, which requires monthly pregnancy testing for females.

Ancillary Treatments

What about physical methods used to treat acne? Again, please remember not to pop pimples or further manipulate active acne lesions. Extraction of open comedones (blackheads) can be accomplished using a comedone extractor. This instrument features an open loop that is placed over the blackened pore, allowing the contents to be expressed when firm pressure is applied. Comedone expression has minimal influence on the course of acne. The widened pore will reaccumulate its blackened contents within a month's time; however, many persons obtain cosmetic benefit from this procedure and welcome the removal of these unsightly black dots.

Lasers, IPL (intense pulsed light), and blue and red light sources are used by some clinicians to treat acne. Such interventions, of varying cost and not covered by insurance, may lessen the need for oral antibiotics. The verdict is still out as to their overall effectiveness.

Persons who develop cysts and larger reddened pimples often benefit from the injection of a steroid solution (Kenalog) directly into each lesion. This medication promotes resolution and helps prevent subsequent scarring.

SCARRING

What can be done for those already scarred by acne? Dermatologists and plastic surgeons possess several tools for the correction of scarring, including dermal filler implants, dermabrasion (mechanical sanding), and lasers. Which procedure(s) to use depends on a number of factors, including the extent and depth of scarring. More superficial scars may respond to a topical retinoid applied on a long-term basis. Shallow, concave, pliable scars respond to dermal filler injection. Satisfactory results have been reported with fractional lasers and a procedure termed *microneedling*, which utilizes needle sticks into the dermis to stimulate collagen production. Keep in mind that although 100 percent correction is unlikely, some degree of improvement may be achieved. Often, the changes are dramatic.

In summary, the goal of acne therapy is to clear up existing blemishes and prevent new ones from appearing. Mild acne may respond to topical therapy with over-the-counter preparations containing benzoyl peroxide, sulfur derivatives, or salicylic acid. However, if these measures fail, consultation with a dermatologist is prudent. Two or more different medications are commonly employed simultaneously. Be patient; acne does not clear up overnight. One should always give a new regimen a minimum of four weeks for visible results. Persons with moderate to severe acne unresponsive to conventional oral therapies should strongly consider isotretinoin, which, for many, is a miracle drug.

Acne is a cosmetically disfiguring ailment. If left untreated, the condition may lead to physical and emotional scarring. Today acne is controllable, and many cases may be cured.

16

Rosacea and Perioral Dermatitis

ROSACEA AND PERIORAL DERMATITIS ARE TWO FACIAL DISORDERS THAT affect women in greater frequency than men. Both are striking causes of a red face.

ROSACEA

Rosacea begins insidiously, often as a prominent, evanescent facial flush. The rosy condition may involve only the lower half of the nose or may spread to cover the so-called blush zone (the cheeks, forehead, and chin). The bouts of redness gradually become more frequent and intense, leading to persistent changes in skin color. Rosacea may be accompanied by crops of inflamed pus-filled pimples (papulopustular variant).

Rosacea affects more than fourteen million Americans. The condition occurs most commonly in fair-skinned women who characteristically develop intense redness following brief sun exposure. A severe form of rosacea affects men. Medically termed *rhinophyma*, the disorder is characterized by uneven, progressive nasal swelling (the W. C. Fields nose), leading to significant cosmetic deformity.

Rosacea can also involve the eyes. Persons with ocular rosacea may experience itching, stinging, dryness, foreign-body sensation, and a watery, bloodshot appearance.

Rosacea is aggravated by the ingestion of hot beverages and alcohol, both of which dilate blood vessels and promote facial redness. Extremes in temperature, as well as excessive sunlight, should be avoided. An otherwise harmless microscopic facial mite (called *Demodex*) has been linked to this condition.

Rosacea Trigger Factors	
Sun exposure	Vigorous exercise
Stress	Wind
Alcohol	Hot baths
Caffeine	Cold weather
Spicy foods	Hot beverages

Persons with rosacea should avoid harsh cleansers, toners, and astringents. When outdoors, apply a high-SPF sunscreen. The mainstay of medical treatment for papulopustular rosacea is the oral antibiotic doxycycline. Oracea is a low-dose doxycycline promoted specifically for rosacea. Topical preparations containing the antibiotic metronidazole (Metrogel, Noritate) may prove useful for treatment of both acute flares and long-term maintenance, as may sulfur-containing compounds (Avar, Klaron, Sulfacet-R) and medications containing azelaic acid (Azelex, Finacea). In 2014, the topical cream Soolantra (1 percent ivermectin) was approved to treat rosacea; this medication reduces colonization of the *Demodex* mite. In 2022, Epsolay was approved to treat papulopustular rosacea. This medication contains encapsulated benzoyl peroxide

Redness associated with rosacea may be lessened with a green-tinted foundation applied underneath one that is skin-toned. The prescription medications Mirvaso gel (brimonidine) and Rhofade cream (oxymetazoline) are approved to treat rosacea-associated redness. Not all people respond, and some experience side effects, such as skin irritation. Treatments of choice for dilated blood vessels accompanying rosacea are specific vascular lasers or IPL (intense pulsed light). Both are simple office procedures with the primary downside of temporary bruising.

PERIORAL DERMATITIS

Perioral dermatitis is a facial condition that primarily affects women in the twenty- to forty-year age group. The problem has become increasingly more common over the past decade.

Tiny red pimples and pustules, as well as dryness and scaling around the mouth and on the chin, characterize perioral dermatitis. Occasional burning or itching may be experienced.

Perioral dermatitis may last from several weeks to many years. The condition waxes and wanes in intensity, and premenstrual worsening is common. The use of high-potency steroid creams will either cause or exacerbate this facial rash, and such use must be immediately discontinued. Topical medications used to treat this condition include Metrogel (metronidazole) and Elidel (pimecrolimus). Some cases may require oral antibiotic therapy.

17

Eczema
(Atopic Dermatitis)

ATOPIC DERMATITIS, KNOWN TO MOST AS ECZEMA, IS A COMMON SKIN disease that affects more than thirty million people in the United States. Atopic dermatitis ranks among the ten most common skin conditions treated by dermatologists. The incidence of this disorder is increasing, and it affects nearly 10 percent of children younger than fourteen years.

Eczema may appear in early childhood, often by the age of four months. The face, scalp, neck, and diaper areas are most frequently involved. These sites, especially the cheeks, become red and scaly. Itching is severe, and the infant may literally tear apart his or her skin, which can lead to bleeding sores and secondary infection. In most cases, itching precedes the appearance of the rash; thus, eczema is commonly referred to as "the itch that rashes." As the child ages, the disorder tends to localize to the back of the neck, behind the elbows and knees, and on the wrists and ankles. The involved sites are dry and thickened and demonstrate accentuation of the normal skin creases (termed *lichenification*).

Most persons with atopic dermatitis experience clearing of the disorder in their late twenties, and by age thirty, a large number are free of disease. In some adults, atopic dermatitis may localize to the hands and feet or may arise as circular, dry, scaling patches termed *nummular eczema*. Eczema at any age is characterized by itching of varying degrees.

The cause of atopic dermatitis is not fully understood. Hay fever and asthma are associated with this condition. Heredity certainly plays an important role, as nearly 70 percent of atopic dermatitis patients have at least one other family member with eczema, hay fever, or asthma. Diet (food allergy) was thought to cause or aggravate the disorder, but this is unlikely, except perhaps in the very early infantile stage. Atopic dermatitis has been linked to chronic inflammation perpetuated by inflammatory proteins called cytokines and to deficiency of hydrating proteins (filaggrins) in the stratum corneum. Bacterial colonization of the skin also plays a role.

Treatment of atopic dermatitis centers on control of the itching, rash, and underlying inflammatory component. Always be mindful that the more one scratches, the worse the disorder becomes and the longer it takes to heal.

Persons with atopic dermatitis should avoid factors that aggravate sensitive skin. Fingernails, especially those of infants, are best trimmed as short as possible to avoid digging and tearing. Clothing should be soft, loose-fitting, and preferably made of cotton; wool and irritating synthetics are best not worn. Overbathing and the use of harsh soaps contribute to skin dryness. Mild, moisturizing soaps and lubricating bath oils are recommended. Moisturizers should be applied to the skin on a regular and frequent basis. Ointments, such as Vaseline and Aquaphor, provide superior lubrication but may be too greasy for some. Creams are less greasy, and those infused with lipids and ceramides are particularly helpful. Leading brands include Aveeno, CeraVe, Cetaphil, and Eucerin.

Individuals with persistent eczema warrant medical care. Topical agents are a mainstay therapy for control of mild to moderate cases and include steroid ointments and creams as well as the calcineurin inhibitors Elidel cream (pimecrolimus) and Protopic ointment (tacrolimus), which have been in use for more than two decades. Eucrisa cream (crisaborole) was approved in 2016 to treat mild to moderate eczema and can be used by individuals three months or older. The JAK inhibitor Opzelura (ruxolitinib) was approved to treat mild to moderate atopic dermatitis in 2021. Elidel, Eucrisa, Opzelura, and Protopic are safe to use on the face and groin, problematic areas for steroids. Oral antihistamines are commonly recommended but of minimal value. A number of antibacterial sprays containing hypochlorous acid (e.g., Levicyn, SkinSmart) decrease surface bacteria and are antipruritic (anti-itch). Additional therapies include ultraviolet light (narrow-band UVB) and, for more severe cases, oral medications, including prednisone, methotrexate, and cyclosporine. A topical medication approved for psoriasis, Vtama (tapinarof), is pending FDA approval to treat eczema.

The approval of Dupixent (dupilumab) in 2017 revolutionized the treatment of eczema. This drug was the first to target specific inflammatory proteins (IL-4 and IL-13) associated with this condition. Dupixent is injected under the skin every two weeks and may take several months for maximal effect. No bloodwork is required prior to or during treatment, and the medication may be used in children as young as six months of age. Some patients develop eye irritation (conjunctivitis), which can necessitate discontinuation. A similar injectable agent, Adbry (tralokinumab), targets IL-13 and was approved in 2021. Yet another IL-13 blocker (lebrikizumab) is pending FDA approval, soon to be followed by the IL-31 blocker nemolizumab.

In 2022, two new agents were approved as treatment for moderate to severe eczema: Cibinqo (abrocitinib) and Rinvoq (upadacitinib). These inhibit a pathway called JAK-STAT, which also plays a key role in the causation of eczema. Cibinqo and Rinvoq are taken daily in pill form and act much faster than the IL-4 and IL-13 inhibitors. Indeed, relief from itch may be noted days after the first dose. Both medications require blood work and carry black-box warnings mandated by the FDA. These include potential risk for serious infection, blood clots, and heart disease, although to date, the risk appears low.

18

Irritant and
Contact Dermatitis

INFLAMMATION OF THE SKIN THAT FOLLOWS DIRECT EXPOSURE TO AN external agent may result from two different mechanisms. In some instances, referred to as irritant dermatitis, a substance physically damages the skin. With contact allergy, a substance triggers an allergic reaction.

IRRITANT DERMATITIS

Industrial workers, food handlers, bartenders, and homemakers frequently suffer from irritant dermatitis of the hands. Exposure to harsh soaps, detergents, and solvents leads to chapping and irritation with repeated use. Excess moisture promotes irritation by increasing the penetration of these substances. Initially, the affected areas (most often the fingers, hands, wrists, and forearms) become red and itchy. Severe dryness, thickening, and cracking result from long-standing exposure, a condition known colloquially as *dishpan hands*.

Treatment of irritant dermatitis involves protection of the involved areas. Strict avoidance of excess heat, moisture, harsh soaps, and detergents is essential. Those affected should avoid unnecessary wetting of the hands. As irritant dermatitis can begin in the moist environment under rings that trap soap and chemicals, rings should be removed before wet work. Specially formulated barrier-protectant emollients help to insulate the skin from environmental damage. Examples include Gloves in a Bottle, O'Keefe's Working Hands, and Proteque.

When washing the hands, use lukewarm water and, if possible, a mild cleanser, such as Aquanil, CeraVe, Cetaphil, or baby soap. Cleansers should be used sparingly, and the hands should be thoroughly rinsed. Carefully dry with a clean towel. Plastic gloves or lined rubber gloves should be worn when washing dishes and clothes, when peeling or squeezing citrus fruits, and when in contact with harsh chemicals. Gloves should not be worn for more than twenty minutes at one time. If water enters the glove, remove it immediately.

Affected hands should be lubricated with a skin cream or lotion several times during the day. Prescription steroid creams may be required in more severe cases.

COSMETIC AND SKIN-CARE PRODUCT ALLERGY

Teenagers and adults often use several different cosmetic products daily. An allergy to a cosmetic or skin-care product manifests as redness, swelling, and itching wherever that substance comes into contact with the skin. If the offending cosmetic is a hair dye, irritated skin will be noted around the ears and along the hairline. An allergy to eye makeup results in swelling and scaling around the eyes, and an allergic response to perfume or cologne will occur at sites of application.

One may use a skin-care product for years without problem and then suddenly become allergic to an ingredient. For this reason, always consider an allergic reaction whenever inflammation of the skin develops in an area of topical application.

If an allergic reaction is suspected, discontinue the potential allergen. Should the reaction subside, assume that this product contains the offending agent. If in doubt, a potential culprit may be applied daily to the same area of the arm, which should then be checked for signs of an allergic response (usually redness). Identification of specific chemicals is accomplished by a procedure called patch testing. Potential allergens are placed on the skin under an adhesive covering, kept in place for forty-eight hours, and then analyzed for redness and swelling.

Additional information on potential allergens follows:

Cosmetic Allergy: Common Culprits

Fragrances: Hundreds of different fragrances are used in products such as perfumes, shampoos, soaps, deodorants, and moisturizers. Even products labeled *unscented* may contain masking fragrances. The area around the eyes is particularly sensitive. When a perfumed spray is involved, redness and itching of the neck are classic as well.

Preservatives: Preservatives are used to extend the life of products and are the second most common cause of contact dermatitis to cosmetics. Ingredients linked to preservative allergic reactions include quaternium-15, parabens, and thimerosal.

Hair dyes: Ingredient labels found on hair dyes warn users to regularly test for allergic reaction prior to use. The most common allergen is phenylenediamine (PPD), the key ingredient in permanent hair dye. Allergic reactions may occur on the forehead and neck before affecting the scalp. PPD is also a commonly found ingredient in black henna temporary tattoos.

Nail products: Allergic reactions to nail polish and acrylic nails may present as redness and swelling about the nail. Touching the face and eyelids with the fingertips can induce a reaction at these sites as well. Causative chemicals include formaldehyde-based resins and acrylates.

JEWELRY ALLERGY

Allergic reactions to jewelry are not uncommon. Indeed, nearly one out of every ten females is sensitive to nickel. People with a nickel allergy develop redness, scaling, and itching wherever this metal comes into contact with the body. Common sites include the earlobes (from earrings), upper chest and back (from bra straps), waistline (from belt buckles), and wrists (from watchbands or bracelets). Nickel allergy is on the rise in part due to the popularity of body piercings and the ubiquitous presence of this metal. Nickel has been designated a past Allergen of the Year by the North American Contact Dermatitis Group.

Once a nickel allergy develops, the sensitivity persists indefinitely. Those affected should avoid prolonged contact with this metal. The chemical solution dimethylglyoxime may be applied to wearable metal to assay for the presence of nickel. Sterling silver, gold, and platinum earrings may be worn, but chances are good that costume and gold-plated jewelry contain nickel.

PLANT ALLERGY

The most common plant allergy is due to poison ivy. Other offenders include poison oak, sumac, and the mango plant. All contain the same irritating chemicals, and all can produce itchy eruptions.

Plant dermatitis follows exposure of a body part to the leaves of an offending plant or to materials that have been in close contact with the plant, such as animal fur or clothing. A rash appears at the sites of exposure after a twenty-four-hour to one-week delay. Fluid-filled blisters arise in patches and streaks, and these are usually quite itchy.

The best way to prevent allergic dermatitis is through avoidance. Persons susceptible to poison plant allergy (this includes about 60 percent of the population) should be familiar with these plants and remain vigilant when gardening, camping, and engaging in other outdoor activities. When walking in wooded areas, wear pants, long-sleeved shirts, and socks. Poison ivy plants may be physically removed (wear gloves!) or chemically destroyed. Exposed skin should be thoroughly washed within fifteen minutes to avoid penetration of the noxious plant chemical. Specific barrier creams, such as Ivy Block and IvyX, may afford adequate protection when applied prior to exposure.

Mild cases of allergic dermatitis respond to drying compounds, such as calamine lotion and oatmeal baths. Over-the-counter hydrocortisone relieves itch. Severe cases are best managed by a physician. Oral desensitization to prevent poison ivy allergy is not recommended.

LATEX ALLERGY

Latex is a compound synthesized from the rubber tree. The use of gloves made with latex markedly increased with concern of contracting blood-borne diseases, such as hepatitis and AIDS. This increase in use was paralleled by an increase in allergic reactions. Latex allergy affects up to 2 percent of Americans and is most frequently encountered in health-care workers.

The most common reaction to latex is either irritant or allergic dermatitis, generally localized to sites of exposure, mainly the hands. Severe latex allergy can cause constriction of the airways (anaphylaxis) and death from airway closure.

Although specific allergy tests are available, most cases of latex allergy are diagnosed by history. The cornerstone of management is strict avoidance of latex. Use of latex-free gloves is mandatory for sensitive individuals, as are recognition and avoidance of other products that may contain latex, such as rubber bands, balloons, and condoms.

19

Psoriasis

PSORIASIS IS A COMMON DISORDER AFFECTING UP TO 3 PERCENT OF THE US population. The condition often has a profound effect on quality of life. In a study conducted by the National Psoriasis Foundation, more than 60 percent of psoriasis patients expressed feelings of self-consciousness.

Classic psoriasis is characterized by red patches covered with a silvery, adherent scale. Any body part may be affected, but the most common sites are the elbows, knees, scalp, genitals, and lower back. Psoriasis can affect the nails, leading to tiny pits, discoloration, or marked thickening and distortion. Approximately 15 percent of psoriasis sufferers develop arthritis, which ranges in intensity from mild to crippling.

Psoriasis frequently begins in young adulthood, although childhood cases do occur. The course of the disorder is variable. In the summer months, the condition may improve, particularly after sun exposure. Worsening may follow a long illness or a period of stress.

The cause of psoriasis is unknown, although abnormalities of the immune system play a seminal role. Heredity is also a factor, and people with close relatives who have psoriasis are more likely to develop the condition. Until the past decade, psoriasis was considered a disease mainly confined to the skin and joints. Large studies have confirmed that persons with psoriasis are at increased risk of developing high blood pressure, elevated blood fat levels, diabetes, and myocardial infarction (heart attack). Psoriatic patients have a higher rate of obesity, which certainly contributes to these comorbidities, but evidence is accumulating that the chronic inflammation associated with psoriasis also adversely affects the heart and blood vessels.

To date, psoriasis is not curable, but the majority of cases can be adequately controlled. For some, complete clearance is achievable. Topical therapies are the mainstay of treatment for mild disease. Topical steroids are available in a variety of forms, including ointments, creams, lotions, gels, sprays, and foams, of which the most potent are clobetasol (Impoyz, Temovate), betamethasone (Diprolene), and halobetasol (Halog). Prolonged use may lead to thinning of the skin. The vitamin A derivative tazarotene (Tazorac) is FDA approved to treat psoriasis, as are vitamin D derivatives (Dovonex, Vectical). Tar shampoo (e.g., DHS, Tarsum, T/Gel) is a useful add-on for scalp psoriasis. In 2022, the FDA approved two nonsteroidal topical medications to treat psoriasis: Vtama (tapinarof) and Zoryve (roflumilast). Both are applied daily and may be used on areas where topical steroids are not advisable, such as the face, armpits, and groin.

Natural and artificial ultraviolet light improve many cases of psoriasis. Narrow-band UVB therapy requires a light box and is considered a first-line therapeutic option. Treatments are ideally administered three times per week, and an average of thirty sessions is required to achieve maximum improvement. A study published in 2023 confirmed that home UVB machines provide cost-effective treatment, although many insurance companies will not cover their purchase. The excimer laser is approved by the FDA to treat psoriasis and emits a more concentrated beam of light. Fewer sessions are required, and some insurance companies may approve coverage.

Three oral therapies have been used for decades to treat moderate to severe psoriasis: acitretin, cyclosporine, and methotrexate.

The oral retinoid acitretin (Soriatane) is a potent derivative of vitamin A. Periodic blood testing is prudent, as this drug can raise the level of circulating triglycerides (fats). Like isotretinoin (used to treat acne), the drug is teratogenic (may cause birth defects) and must be used with extreme caution in females of childbearing age and never by pregnant females.

The response to cyclosporine (Neoral, Sandimmune) may be rapid, sometimes occurring within two weeks. The drug is taken daily and works by suppressing certain aspects of the immune system. Cyclosporine may raise blood pressure and serum lipid levels. It can also decrease kidney function, necessitating periodic laboratory monitoring.

Methotrexate is used to treat both psoriasis and psoriatic arthritis. An advantage of methotrexate is that the entire dose is taken once weekly. A favorable response is usually noted within six weeks. Methotrexate can induce nausea, a low white blood cell count, and liver damage. Periodic blood testing is mandatory. A liver biopsy may be recommended after prolonged use. Methotrexate should never be used by pregnant females or anyone who drinks excessive alcohol.

The year 2004 marked a revolution in the treatment of psoriasis with FDA approval of Enbrel (Etanercept) to treat this condition. Enbrel is classified as a biologic, which is a substance produced by human or animal protein rather than chemicals. All biologics are administered by injection, and these have proven to be miracle drugs for many patients, markedly improving or even clearing skin, nail, and scalp disease. They're considered safer and more efficacious than traditional systemic therapies. Their greatest drawback is high cost.

Biologics are classified by the way they block inflammatory agents linked to psoriasis. There's no need to dwell on specifics, so here is a quick review. Inflammatory mediators of psoriasis fall into several classes: TNF alpha, interleukin 17, and interleukins 12 and 23. TNF alpha inhibitors include Cimzia (certolizumab), Enbrel (etanercept), Humira (adalimumab), and Remicade (infliximab). All are self-injected under the skin, similar to insulin, except for Remicade, which is administered through a vein. TNF alpha inhibitors are also approved to treat psoriatic arthritis. IL-23 inhibitors are Ilumya (tildrakizumab), Skyrizi (risankizumab), Stelara (ustekinumab, which also blocks IL-12), and Tremfya (guselkumab). The latter three are approved to treat psoriatic arthritis. IL-17 inhibitors are Bimzelx (bimekizumab), approved in 2023; Cosentyx (secukinumab); Siliq (brodalumab); and Taltz (ixekizumab). IL-17 inhibitors are best avoided by patients with a history of gastrointestinal ailments. Cosentyx and Taltz are also approved to treat psoriatic arthritis. Cosentyx, Enbrel, Stelara, and Taltz are approved to treat children with psoriasis.

Prior to the start of any biologic, a patient requires testing for tuberculosis. Dosing is variable. For example, Enbrel is administered weekly; Tremfya every two months; and Ilumya, Skyrizi, and Stelara every three months. Efficacy varies; the least effective and most inconvenient dosing is Enbrel, which is now primarily used to treat psoriatic arthritis and children. All biologics carry the warning of a potential increased risk for infection.

Otezla (apremilast) was approved to treat psoriasis and psoriatic arthritis in 2014. This drug is taken by mouth twice daily. No blood work is required. Diarrhea is a side effect that may limit use. Another oral agent, Sotyktu, was approved in 2022 to treat psoriasis. It's taken once daily, and limited blood work is required. Sotyktu has better efficacy than Otezla but not as high as several of the biologics.

As noted, biologics are very expensive. Coverage of a particular drug may be dictated by one's insurance company rather than the preference of a medical provider. Entering the biologic space are biosimilars, less expensive options with similar potency and safety. These agents will lower cost and, by doing so, are expected to provide greater access to therapy.

Psoriasis is a lifelong condition that affects millions of Americans. Long-term treatment is required for management. Significant medical advances that target immune pathways responsible for disease ensure that nearly everyone with psoriasis will improve. Some individuals with severe, debilitating disease can even achieve 100 percent clearance. Dermatology practices specialize in therapeutic options designed to control this disorder, and consultation is highly recommended. Individuals with psoriasis are also encouraged to contact the National Psoriasis Foundation (psoriasis.org) and the American Academy of Dermatology (aad.org).

20

Common Skin Infections

FUNGAL AND YEAST INFECTIONS

Fungi and yeast all too often view our skin as fertile pasture. When these organisms take root, their presence is made known in a variety of ways, some decidedly more unpleasant than others. Yeast inhabits skin and mucous membranes, and fungi colonize virtually everywhere, including the hair and nails. The many varied conditions caused by fungi and yeast follow.

TINEA

Grandparents can remember classmates in elementary school sent home because of ringworm. Few knew exactly what ringworm was, but it sounded horrible.

What is ringworm? Certainly not a worm! Ringworm is a contagious disorder of the skin or hair caused by a fungal infection. A more appropriate name is tinea.

Fungal infection of the scalp is termed *tinea capitis*. As a rule, fungi only infect the scalps of preadolescents, because at puberty, scalp oil glands secrete substances that inhibit their growth. In other words, immunity to most fungal scalp infections is in place by the time one reaches junior high school.

Patchy areas of hair loss containing broken, fragmented hairs characterize tinea capitis. In more severe cases, these areas may contain scales and even pus-filled pimples. Because scalp tinea is contagious to other children and may lead to permanent hair loss, treatment should commence as soon as the diagnosis is made. Oral therapy with either griseofulvin or terbinafine (Lamisil) is required for cure.

Tinea elsewhere, although more common in children, may also occur in adults. Body ringworm (tinea corporis) is characterized by scaly, circular red patches that frequently itch. These patches characteristically have clearer centers, hence the ringlike appearance. Nonprescription creams containing clotrimazole (Lotrimin), miconazole (Micatin), and terbinafine (Lamisil) are curative, although more extensive cases may require oral antifungal therapy as well.

ATHLETE'S FOOT: TINEA PEDIS

Athlete's foot (tinea pedis) is one of the most common fungal infections. Unlike body and scalp ringworm, this disorder is generally an ailment of adult life. You don't have to be an athlete to get athlete's foot, but it sure helps. Fungi love sweaty feet, and they thrive on moist shower floors.

A fungal infection of the feet is characterized by itching, redness, and scaling. Severe cases may be accompanied by blisters. The condition most commonly occurs between the toes and may spread to the soles.

Prevention and treatment of athlete's foot entail minimizing excess heat and perspiration. Shoes that permit ventilation are preferred. Leather shoes and sandals are the best; plastic shoes and sneakers are the worst. The feet should be thoroughly dried after bathing and then coated with a drying powder (e.g., Desenex, Zeasorb) before socks are worn. Mild to moderate cases can be controlled with antifungal creams; more severe cases may require oral antifungal therapy.

JOCK ITCH: TINEA CRURIS

Tinea of the groin (tinea cruris) affects primarily men, especially in the summer months. Predisposing factors are moisture retention, heat, friction, and obesity. An itchy red rash of the upper thighs and/or backside characterizes tinea cruris.

Avoidance of tight, restrictive underclothing aids in the prevention and treatment. Drying powders that soak up excess moisture are also helpful. Cure is achieved with antifungal creams, although recurrence is common.

NAIL INFECTIONS

Fungal infection of the nails (onychomycosis) begins at the free margins and sides and results in yellowish discoloration, increased thickness, and brittleness. Toenails are more frequently involved than fingernails. The condition affects tens of millions of Americans, most after the age of forty.

Nail fungal infections may prove cosmetically disfiguring, given the distortion and color changes. Some may be painful and interfere with walking. The condition is difficult to treat, requiring many weeks of oral antifungal therapy (usually terbinafine). About 60 percent of those treated will be cured. Topical therapy (Jublia, Kerydin, and Penlac solutions) may prevent worsening but has a much lower cure rate. Painful toenails can be surgically removed.

TINEA VERSICOLOR

Ever look in the mirror and discover that your back and chest have become dotted with multiple scaling, discolored patches? These spots are likely tinea versicolor.

Tinea versicolor ranks among the most common of all skin disorders. This noncontagious condition is caused by a ubiquitous yeast-like organism that can breach the outermost layer of skin, resulting in either light or dark flat areas containing fine scale. Tinea versicolor is most common in teenagers and young adults and is rare in children and senior citizens. Itching is mild, if at all. The infection is most apparent in the summer months, as involved skin does not tan after sun exposure.

Tinea versicolor may respond to a variety of different compounds, including daily applications of selenium sulfide lotion (Excel, Selsun), ketoconazole shampoo (Nizoral), or a wide range of antifungal creams. More extensive cases are treated with fluconazole (Diflucan). The discoloration may take months to normalize, and recurrence is common.

YEAST VAGINITIS

Yeast infection of the mucous membranes is called candidiasis or moniliasis. Vaginal yeast infections often occur during pregnancy and in diabetics. Certain antibiotics (especially tetracycline) and birth control pills may predispose to yeast overgrowth.

Candidiasis is characterized by a thin white discharge accompanied by severe itching. The condition is treated with antifungal creams, vaginal inserts, and oral antiyeast medications, such as fluconazole. Women with recurrent yeast infections warrant testing for diabetes.

THRUSH: ORAL CANDIDIASIS

Oral thrush results from yeast overgrowth within the mouth and presents with creamy to whitish patches affecting the tongue and inner cheeks. Scraping these sites can result in slight bleeding. This condition is most common in babies, toddlers, and older adults. Risk factors in adults include uncontrolled diabetes; cancer therapies, including chemotherapy and radiation; HIV; and oral antibiotics. Sore mouth and loss of taste are common symptoms.

Thrush is usually treated with a topical therapy, such as nystatin, available as a pastille, mouthwash, and oral suspension used several times daily for two weeks. An alternative therapy is clotrimazole troches (Mycelex). Refractory cases warrant oral therapy with fluconazole (Diflucan).

PARONYCHIA

A paronychia is a swelling of the finger just below the nail. Many cases are associated with yeast infection. The tissue adjacent to the nail becomes red, swollen, and tender to the touch.

Paronychias are more common in women and frequently afflict persons who have their hands in and out of water, such as homemakers, bartenders, and hairdressers. Avoidance of moisture and irritants is usually necessary for complete cure. Gloves should be worn to protect the hands if wet work cannot be curtailed. Cuticles must not be unduly manipulated, and nail cosmetics are best avoided. Medical treatment consists of the application of antibacterial, antiyeast, and/or anti-inflammatory creams or solutions two to three times daily.

INTERTRIGO

The inflammation that occurs wherever skin surfaces rub against each other is called intertrigo. The favored sites are the groin, under the arms and breasts, the buttocks, and between the toes. Contributing factors besides friction are heat, moisture, and sweat retention. Overweight persons are prone to developing intertrigo.

Intertrigo is characterized by redness, maceration, and irritation of the affected areas. In severe cases, the skin may weep and crack open.

Intertrigo is caused by a mixture of fungi, yeast, and bacteria. Treatment entails thorough cleansing and drying of the involved sites. The application of topical anti-yeast and/or antibacterial creams helps to resolve the condition. Use of medicated powders may prevent reoccurrence. Obese persons are urged to lose weight.

Bacterial Infections

IMPETIGO

An enormous number of bacteria reside on the skin's surface (four million microbes on just the hands!). Usually, these germs peacefully coexist with the human host, but on occasion, they invade beneath the skin and cause disease. Impetigo is a contagious infection caused by either the streptococcus or the staphylococcus bacterium. Preschool and school-age children are most commonly affected.

Impetigo begins as a small, itchy reddish area that rapidly develops pus-filled pimples exuding a sticky fluid. Within one to two days, a thick, adherent golden-yellow crust forms over the region. The face is the most common location, especially around the chin and nose. If neglected, the infection may spread to other parts of the body.

Warm water soaks to the affected sites, followed by application of an antibacterial ointment, such as mupirocin, will successfully treat most cases. The patient and close contacts should wash daily with an antibacterial soap. Extensive, rapidly spreading cases require antibiotics taken by mouth and should be medically evaluated. Adequate therapy quickly resolves the infection and prevents more serious consequences.

CELLULITIS

Cellulitis is an acute bacterial infection that manifests as a hot, well-defined, tender red area of skin. The most common causative agents are streptococcal and staphylococcal germs, which enter the skin secondary to minor trauma, such as a scratch or insect bite. Growth and invasion of bacteria produce inflammation, tenderness, warmth, and redness. The disorder is not contagious. Persons with diabetes are prone to developing this condition.

All cases of cellulitis should be evaluated by a health-care provider. Hot compresses and oral antibiotics usually result in prompt resolution; if not, or if the condition is accompanied by elevated temperature, blood culture may be ordered to rule out spread of the infection.

FLESH-EATING BACTERIA: NECROTIZING FASCIITIS

Necrotizing fasciitis is an uncommon but serious bacterial infection that destroys skin along with fat and muscle beneath it. The damage is the result of toxins secreted by the bacteria.

Most persons who acquire the disease are in good health. The portal of entry may be as trivial as a small nick. Within twenty-four to thirty-six hours, the injured site worsens. Symptoms may include fever, chills, and excruciating pain. Immediate medical care and hospitalization are mandatory. Surgical debridement and IV antibiotics can be lifesaving; some 30 percent of persons who contract necrotizing fasciitis die from the disease.

BOILS

A boil is a localized skin infection caused by the staphylococcus germ. The involved area develops a raised red sore that is filled with pus. The sore is often sensitive to light touch. The skin thins out in the center, and a whitish-yellow point forms. This ruptures within two to four days, spilling out the enclosed pus.

Boils may form almost anywhere on the body but are most commonly encountered on sites of hair-bearing skin subject to friction and maceration, such as the buttocks, neck, face, underarms, and thighs. Boils may be spread from person to person by close contact. Hence, athletes participating in contact sports, such as football and wrestling, are prone to boils. Staphylococcal infections are readily passed to sex partners and to members of the same household.

Never squeeze a boil! Squeezing and picking at sores may spread the infection and leave scars. Small boils are best treated with hot, moist compresses applied three to four times a day. The area should be frequently washed with a strong antibacterial soap, such as Dial or Safeguard. When the boil begins to drain, pus should be removed as it forms and not allowed to contaminate surrounding skin. Towels, linens, and clothing used by a person with a boil should be kept separate until thoroughly washed. Large boils are best drained by a medical provider, who will also determine the need for an oral antibiotic.

MRSA

MRSA stands for *methicillin-resistant staphylococcus aureus*, and it is a growing problem in the United States. Although most cases occur in hospitals or other health-care settings, an increasing percentage are being noted elsewhere, including high schools and colleges (often spread by contact sports, such as wrestling and football). Clinically, lesions start as pimples that may evolve into painful abscesses.

Suspected abscesses should be drained as soon as possible and cultured. Oral antibiotics may be required. The spread of MRSA is best halted by frequent hand washing or use of an alcohol-based sanitizer.

LYME DISEASE

Lyme disease is now the most diagnosed insect-borne disease in the United States, with an estimated 450,000 people treated for this condition each year. The causative organism is transmitted to humans by the bite of a deer tick. The longer an infected tick remains attached to the body, the greater the risk of catching the disease. The first symptom of Lyme disease is usually an expanding red rash that resembles a bull's-eye. This appears one to four weeks after the tick bite and may measure several inches in diameter. The rash is painless and does not itch, but it may be accompanied by fever, chills, and joint pains. As the bacterium multiplies throughout the body, additional symptoms can include fatigue, severe headache, and even facial nerve paralysis (Bell's palsy). Advanced Lyme disease can lead to neurologic deficits and persistent arthritis.

Lyme disease responds to oral antibiotics, which are best started as soon as a diagnosis is made. A specific blood test cannot be relied upon early in the disease. Preventative measures include wearing long sleeves and pants when walking in wooded or grassy areas, using insect repellants containing DEET, and gently removing any tick by using tweezers to pull the creature straight out.

SYPHILIS

Syphilis is a bacterial infection spread by sexual contact. The disease starts as a painless sore (chancre) on the genitals, mouth, or anus a short time after exposure. As sores are painless and in areas not readily visualized, some individuals remain unaware of infection. The chancre resolves within several weeks, soon to be followed by the secondary stage, which usually manifests as a reddened rash of the trunk with involvement of the palms and soles. The rash does not itch. Secondary syphilis too resolves without a trace over time. Treatment with penicillin during either stage is curative. Untreated, syphilis can damage the brain, nerves, and heart. Pregnant females can pass syphilis to their newborns, which can lead to deafness, teeth problems, and deformed noses. Infection with syphilis is confirmed by a blood test.

Both syphilis and congenital syphilis are rising at an alarming rate. Several reasons are cited, including insufficient funding of public health clinics, the stigma over sex, medical provider unfamiliarity with early skin signs, internet dating, and condom fatigue. According to the Centers for Disease Control (CDC), men who have sex with men are one hundred times more likely to be infected than men who have sex with women.

Viral Infections

HERPES SIMPLEX

Herpes simplex is a nasty virus capable of producing blisters on both the lips (cold sores) and the genitals. These sores are painful and unsightly and afflict millions of people each year. The virus is spread to others by intimate contact.

Cold Sore

A cold sore or fever blister is the result of herpes virus localized to the skin in and around the lips. The infection begins with pain or itching, followed by the typical fluid-filled blisters. The sores form a crust and dry up some seven to ten days later. Repeated episodes are commonplace. Sunlight, emotional upset, and illness may awaken the virus and lead to new blisters. Some persons only develop a single episode; others are not as fortunate and develop recurrent blisters once a year or even as frequently as once a month.

Genital Herpes

Chances are good that a painful sore on the genitals is due to herpes simplex infection. This contagious disorder is spread by sexual intercourse and oral sex. The CDC estimates that more than one million people become newly infected each year. It is believed that one in five American adults has been exposed to the virus.

Like the cold sore, genital herpes infection begins with burning or itching, followed by blisters that crust over and finally disappear. Blisters may arise on both male and female genitalia. Many cases, especially in females, are termed *subclinical*—that is, occurring without noticeable signs or symptoms—and some individuals are unaware of infection.

Genital herpes may lead to serious consequences in newborns. A child born to a mother with active lesions at time of delivery runs a high risk of catching the virus when exiting the birth canal. Such infection may prove fatal, necessitating delivery by cesarean section.

To date, herpes is incurable. The oral antiviral medications acyclovir (Zovirax), famciclovir (Famvir), and valacyclovir (Valtrex) diminish episode severity. When taken daily, these medications also lessen the frequency of attacks and the amount of viral shedding between outbreaks. Topical antiviral ointments are much less efficacious. Various other treatment modalities, including lysine pills and dimethyl sulfoxide (DMSO), are without merit. All first episodes of herpes should be evaluated by a clinician to ensure correct diagnosis and adequate counseling.

Herpetic lesions are best kept clean and dry. A topical anesthetic may temporarily relieve the discomfort. The annoying blisters of herpes dry up within a two-week period. Herpes is most contagious when visible lesions are present, and intimate, unprotected contact should be avoided during this period. Between outbreaks of genital herpes, condom use is prudent to prevent transmission.

Persons afflicted with herpes should derive consolation from the natural course of the condition; over time, the number of attacks generally subsides, and episodes diminish in intensity and duration. The disease tends to burn out. Herpes vaccines are currently being tested on human volunteers.

HERPES ZOSTER (SHINGLES)

Herpes zoster, more commonly known as shingles, results in acute, painful blistering eruptions. The same virus that causes chicken pox leads to this condition as well. Following a chicken pox infection, the virus hibernates in nerves under the skin, only to surface as herpes zoster at a future date. Unlike with herpes simplex, a person usually develops herpes zoster only once. Persons with cancer and immunosuppression are at greatest risk.

The onset of shingles is heralded by severe pain in a localized distribution. Because discomfort may precede the rash by some twenty-four hours, early diagnosis is sometimes difficult. Indeed, herpes zoster of the chest is at times misdiagnosed as a heart attack. Once the redness and blisters appear, the nature of the pain becomes apparent.

Complications of herpes zoster are infrequent but serious. Agonizing, persistent pain may localize to the affected area for weeks or months and is referred to as *postherpetic neuralgia*. Elderly persons are at greatest risk of developing this painful sequela, which may be minimized by starting antiviral medication as soon as the rash appears. The zoster virus may also invade the eye and damage vision, necessitating ophthalmologic consultation.

Herpes zoster will arise in more than 10 percent of the population. The disorder becomes increasingly likely with advancing age. The vaccine Shingrix stimulates antibody production and provides strong protection against shingles and postherpetic neuralgia. The vaccine is recommended for most persons aged fifty and older or any adult with a weakened immune system.

MOLLUSCUM CONTAGIOSUM

Molluscum contagiosum is a viral disorder characterized by the appearance of pearly white to flesh-colored papules. Close inspection of each lesion usually reveals a slight depression (umbilication). The disorder is spread by skin-to-skin contact and most commonly occurs in children, with lesions typically involving the face, trunk, and arms. In sexually active adults, molluscum are spread during sexual activity, and the lesions tend to localize to the upper thighs, lower abdomen, and genitals.

Untreated, molluscum may persist for months but will spontaneously clear without scarring. They can be removed in a physician's office by minor surgery (scraping with a curette), liquid nitrogen, or cantharidin, a sticky substance derived from the juice of a blister beetle. Ycanth is a physician-applied cantharidin delivery device approved by the FDA in 2023 to treat molluscum contagiosum. In 2024, the FDA approved the first at-home therapy for molluscum contagiosum: Zelsuvmi (berdazimer) gel.

VIRAL RASH

Several viral diseases are characterized by fever and a typical body rash. The three most common are measles, German measles, and chicken pox.

MEASLES

Measles is a highly contagious disorder that begins much like the common cold, with nasal stuffiness and a dry cough. The skin eruption starts on the face and is accompanied by high fever. The rash spreads downward to involve the neck, trunk, and extremities and reaches its peak in three to five days. Most cases of measles occur in children. Measles is prevented with a vaccine that has been widely distributed for more than fifty years. Resurgence in the United States, fueled in part by COVID fatigue and misinformation spread by antivaxxers, highlights the importance of vaccination.

GERMAN MEASLES

Symptoms associated with German measles (rubella) are usually mild and include headache, fatigue, and slight temperature elevation. Shortly thereafter, a dusky, blotchy red rash appears on the face and rapidly extends to the trunk and extremities. Lymph nodes behind the ears are often enlarged and tender. German measles is only of concern when it occurs in a pregnant woman; rubella in pregnancy leads to eye defects, deafness, and heart malformations in the newborn. As with measles, German measles is prevented with vaccination.

CHICKEN POX

Chicken pox is another once-common infectious disease caused by a virus and characterized by a unique skin eruption. The disease begins with moderate fever and malaise, followed by an itchy rash. The rash starts as pimples that rapidly become filled with fluid. Each is surrounded by a red base; the configuration is likened to dewdrops on a rose petal. Lesions become crusted within four to five days, although new ones may continue to form for about two weeks.

The number of cases of chicken pox has plummeted in the United States since a vaccine was introduced in 1995. Before the vaccine, four million Americans developed the disease each year, and more than ten thousand required hospitalizations. Children should receive the first vaccine dose at twelve to fifteen months of age and a second between ages four and six.

PITYRIASIS ROSEA

Pityriasis rosea is a common skin condition with the highest incidence in adolescents and young adults. Most cases occur in spring and fall. The disorder begins with a single oval lesion covered with a fine scale, which is referred to as the *herald patch*. A few days later, smaller patches arise, especially on the chest and back. On the back, the ovoid lesions follow skin lines and are arranged in a so-called fir tree distribution. Pityriasis rosea rarely affects the face. Itching, if present at all, is usually minimal.

The mainstay of treatment is simple reassurance. All lesions disappear within three to eight weeks. Concern has been raised for pityriasis rosea acquired during pregnancy, which may increase the risk of birth complications and miscarriage.

Stephen M. Schleicher, MD

HIV AND AIDS

AIDS is caused by a virus and transmitted by sexual relations or intravenous drug abuse. *AIDS* stands for *acquired immunodeficiency syndrome*. The virus (HIV) attacks the immune system and, if untreated, leads to debility and death. HIV slowly destroys infection-fighting CD4 T cells in a process that may take years to transform into AIDS. Nearly two million Americans have been diagnosed with HIV. Most cases arise in gay and bisexual men.

The first signs of advancing infection frequently involve the skin. White patches (thrush) may form in the mouth due to yeast overgrowth. Severe, persistent facial and scalp scaling (seborrheic dermatitis) may also accompany HIV. Herpes zoster (shingles) can be triggered by viral infection, and an HIV-positive individual is more prone to a multitude of ordinary and bizarre bacterial, viral, and fungal infections. An uncommon form of skin cancer, Kaposi's sarcoma, is found in association with AIDS and is triggered by a specific virus.

HIV infection is diagnosed by a blood test. In the mid-1990s, AIDS was a leading cause of death in this country, but newer therapies have dramatically improved prognosis, and today HIV has evolved into a chronic but livable condition. Because there is currently no cure or effective vaccine, the key to curbing the spread of HIV is prevention. High-risk individuals can protect against HIV by taking antiviral medications prophylactically, termed *PrEP*. Drugs include Descovy, Truvada, and Apretude.

21

Infestations

SCABIES

SCABIES IS A CONTAGIOUS DISORDER CHARACTERIZED BY ITCHY SKIN. The cause is a tiny mite barely visible as a minuscule speck. The creature is attracted to skin because of the warmth. The mite burrows within the top layer, which results in intense itching that is especially severe at night. Areas commonly affected include the finger webs, wrists, buttocks, penis, and nipples. Burrowing of the mite triggers red scratch marks and punctate bleeding points. The face is rarely involved, except in infants.

Scabies is spread from person to person by direct contact. The condition readily infects other household members, sexual partners, and schoolchildren. Scabies has become epidemic in this country; more than one million Americans each year contract the so-called itch mite.

Scabies is usually diagnosed by the appearance of multiple scratched marks and history of intense itching that is worst at night. Sometimes the burrows of the mite can be seen under a magnifying glass. Scabies can be visualized under a microscope or with an instrument called a dermatoscope.

Scabies is eradicated with topical and/or oral medications. Permethrin-containing cream is applied over the entire body, except the face, for about eight hours and then thoroughly washed off. Retreatment in seven to ten days is necessary. Lesions will clear in some two to three weeks. The oral medication ivermectin will also cure most cases of scabies. Again, two doses approximately one week apart are required. Due to the increase in resistant strains, many clinicians institute therapy with both oral and topical agents simultaneously.

LICE

Lice are bloodsucking insects that infest the scalp, body, and genital areas.

The scalp louse lays some three hundred eggs, each cemented to a hair shaft. Newborn lice must feed within twenty-four hours, or they will perish. Head lice usually affect children and are readily transferred among classmates; millions of schoolchildren are affected each year. Infestation triggers intense itching and scratching, which leads to open sores. Close examination reveals tiny white specks (nits) glued to the hair shaft.

Body lice may be transmitted by close contact or by wearing infested garments. The adult louse feeds on the skin and lives within the seams of clothing. Most cases are associated with dirty, unsanitary living conditions.

Crab lice affect the hairy genital regions. They are spread by sexual contact and infest more than one million Americans on a yearly basis. Crab lice result in ferocious itching of the genitals, which is especially severe at night. On close examination, the tiny louse may be seen as a brownish speck at the base of a pubic hair. Their eggs, or nits, are visible as small dots affixed to the hairs.

Lice are destroyed with medicated creams, lotions, or shampoos. Resistance is an emerging problem with head lice. First-line therapy includes over-the-counter shampoos, such as Rid or Nix. Prescription medications are available as well (Ovide, Sklice, Ulesfia lotion). Given that the nits hatch in several days, repeat treatment is recommended with most therapies. Removal of nits is often impractical and not necessary but can be accomplished using special louse combs. Children with lice or their eggs do not need to be sent home from school.

BEDBUGS

Bedbugs are on the rise, sparing no socioeconomic group. Reasons include increased travel (hitchhiking in luggage), immigration, and resistance to common insecticides. Although commonly associated with poverty and uncleanliness, the nasty critters occasionally make headlines by setting up residence in some of the poshest hotels.

A bedbug bite goes unnoticed, and intense itching only develops later; this is the result of an allergic reaction. Often, the bites are arranged in groups of three, appetizingly referred to as "breakfast, lunch, and dinner." Sometimes the tiny buggers can be seen; wake up in the middle of the night, and shine a flashlight on the bedsheets. The insects are small and flat, less than one-quarter of an inch in diameter. Infestation can also be recognized by the presence of red-brown specks (bedbug excrement) on sheets and mattress seams. The bugs can also live in cracks and crevices and under baseboards. Bedbugs avoid light and roam at night, drawn to a human host by body heat. They dine (suck blood) for five to ten minutes, during which time their body weight swells some 200 percent. Bedbugs, fortunately, do not transmit diseases. But they do transmit fear and loathing and are responsible for many sleepless nights.

Treating bedbug bites is easy. A topical steroid cream and an oral antihistamine will do the trick. Ridding one's residence of these nasty critters is the hard part, as bedbugs can survive for up to a year after a single meal. Scrub infested areas with a stiff brush, and vacuum cracks and crevices. Use of special mattress bags will entomb the bugs and eventually kill them. Heat destroys bedbugs and their eggs, so items such as clothes, bedding, and stuffed animals are best placed in a clothes dryer set on the highest setting for at least twenty minutes. Bug bombs are not effective. A professional exterminator is often the best option and may require more than one visit.

22

Hives

SURELY ALL OF US KNOW SOMEONE WHO HAS BROKEN OUT IN HIVES after ingesting a certain food or medicine. The condition is medically termed *urticaria*, and it affects more than 15 percent of the population during their lifespan.

Urticaria begins as a sensation of itching in a localized area. Minutes later, the hive (or wheal) arises, lasting for minutes or hours before vanishing without a trace. Subsequent hives may appear anywhere else on the body, including the lips, mouth, genitals, and eyelids. Some hives may be induced by light pressure applied to the skin (dermatographism). Hives result from fluid leaking out of blood vessels located under the skin's surface. The vessels experience increased permeability secondary to release of the chemical histamine from specialized cells circulating in the bloodstream.

Anaphylaxis is the most serious form of urticaria. The reaction is widespread and severe. The throat and lungs are affected, swelling up and filling with fluid. Breathing becomes labored, and death from asphyxiation can result. Anaphylaxis is a life-threatening medical emergency.

Urticaria is an allergic response most frequently caused by drugs, such as aspirin and penicillin; foods, with the most common being strawberries, shellfish, and peanuts; and insect bites, such as bee stings. In some cases, the allergic agent (allergen) is difficult to track down; for instance, urticaria has been linked to food preservatives and dyes and to infection caused by a parasite. Some persons develop hives when emotionally upset or under stress.

If the cause of hives is not readily apparent, a detailed diary recording every ingested food item and drug (including over-the-counter therapies, such as aspirin) might prove beneficial. Included in this record should be every instance of a new wheal. Reviewing such a diary might help pinpoint the causative allergen.

Those prone to or suffering from hives should avoid ingestion of citrus fruits, shellfish, and certain pain remedies (both over-the-counter and prescription), all of which can cause or potentially worsen this condition. Caution is warranted when taking prescribed antibiotics, most notably penicillin and ampicillin. Notify a physician at the first sign of a rash.

The itching of hives may be relieved by cool-water compresses. Oatmeal and cornstarch baths are soothing. Hives are treated medically with antihistamines, traditionally Benadryl (diphenhydramine) and Atarax (hydroxyzine). These may cause drowsiness, so drive and operate machinery with care. A better option is nonsedating agents, such as Allegra (fexofenadine), Claritin (loratadine), and Zyrtec (cetirizine), all available without prescription. Some acute or persistent cases may also require oral or intramuscular steroids. Xolair (omalizumab) was approved for the treatment of persistent hives in 2014. Classified as a biologic, Xolair is administered through a needle on a monthly basis and tapered or discontinued when the condition improves or resolves.

Persons experiencing wheezing or shortness of breath (anaphylaxis) require epinephrine (adrenaline), which may prove lifesaving. EpiPen and EpiPen Jr are autoinjectors designed for self-administration.

23

Endocrine Disorders

DIABETES

THE INCIDENCE OF DIABETES IS INCREASING AT AN ALARMING RATE, IN large part due to expanding bellies, sedentary lifestyles, and lack of exercise. Diabetes affects more than 6 percent of the US population, and the condition negatively impacts not only the circulatory system and kidneys but also the skin.

Individuals with poorly controlled blood sugar are prone to a variety of skin infections, especially those caused by yeast (candidiasis) and bacteria (mainly staph). Most of these infections respond well to medical therapies but tend to reoccur.

Of particular concern is any infection, abrasion, or ulceration of the lower extremities. Diabetics may experience clogging of veins and arteries (peripheral vascular disease) and nerve damage. Nerve damage leads to loss of sensation in the legs and feet (peripheral neuropathy). With neuropathy, skin injury in a diabetic may not be felt and, hence, is easily overlooked. Even superficial foot injuries are prone to slow healing, infection, and ulceration, A dreaded sequela is gangrene, which signifies death of tissue, a prelude to amputation. Diabetics have a 15 percent lifetime risk of developing lower-extremity ulceration and are advised to have their legs and feet checked on a regular basis.

Diabetics commonly develop dark areas on the lower legs. This benign but unsightly condition is called diabetic dermopathy or shin spots. The rash is not painful and does not itch. It occurs in more than half of diabetics, most frequently in individuals above the age of fifty with long-standing disease. There is no effective treatment, and lesions may persist for years or spontaneously disappear.

A small percentage of diabetics (less than 1 percent) are afflicted with necrobiosis lipoidica diabeticorum. This unsightly condition is characterized by the presence of waxy yellowish-red patches and plaques localized to the lower legs. The disorder is more common in women. Treatment is far from satisfactory, and the lesions, although not painful, may ulcerate. Diabetics may also develop tense blisters of the feet (diabetic bullae), which are caused by increased skin fragility. The blisters usually heal uneventfully. Acanthosis nigricans is a skin condition arising on the neck and underarms. Affected areas develop a distinct, velvety black appearance. Individuals who are diabetic and obese are at greatest risk. The condition is benign but unsightly.

THYROID DISEASE

The thyroid is a hormone-producing gland that resides within the lower neck and plays an important role in the regulation of many body functions. Twenty million Americans have some type of thyroid disorder. Hair, skin, and nails are particularly susceptible to disorders of this gland. The thyroid also interacts with the immune system, and some individuals with chronic hives and vitiligo have antibodies directed against the thyroid.

Too much hormone is produced when the thyroid is overactive. Excess thyroid hormone leads to the condition called hyperthyroidism, which is characterized by sweating, fine shaking (tremor), weight loss, diarrhea, and heart palpitations. Affected individuals tend to feel hot and prefer cold surroundings. The skin becomes smooth, velvety, and moist. Itching can be generalized and persistent. Swelling and discoloration of the ankles, called pretibial myxedema, is also a hallmark of thyroid disease. Fingernails and toenails may become distorted and separate from the nail base. Treatment options for hyperthyroid disease include specific drugs, radioactive iodine, and surgery.

Too little hormone characterizes hypothyroidism. Symptoms include fatigue, weight gain, cold intolerance, and constipation. The skin becomes cold, pale, dry, and coarse. Puffiness about the eyes is common. Nails become rigid and brittle, and hair markedly thins and may fall out in clumps. Wound healing is impaired, and a simple laceration may take longer than normal to heal. Hypothyroidism is treated with thyroid-replacement medication.

Diseases of the thyroid require medical attention and are diagnosed by symptoms, physical examination, and an analysis of circulating hormones in the blood. Both underactive and overactive thyroid disease can affect not only the skin but also the heart and circulatory systems. Some thyroid-induced skin changes may normalize once adequate control is achieved.

24

Autoimmune Diseases

ON OCCASION, THE HUMAN BODY BECOMES CONFUSED AND STARTS rejecting normal tissue. This is the result of antibodies directed against certain body parts. The antibodies are called autoantibodies (*auto* for "self"), and the resultant pathology is called autoimmune disease. Several autoimmune disorders can have profound effects upon the skin.

LUPUS

The autoantibodies associated with lupus may attack many organs, including the kidneys, heart, joints, and central nervous system. Internal involvement represents the most serious form of the disease and is called systemic lupus erythematosus (SLE). Ninety percent of individuals with SLE are females. The classic skin finding is a so-called butterfly rash characterized by a zone of redness and dilated blood vessels affecting the nose and cheeks. The rash may be induced or worsened by exposure to sunlight and indoor tanning. Ultraviolet light can also precipitate internal organ flares, and those with SLE should avoid exposure and, whenever outdoors, apply a broad-spectrum sunscreen of at least SPF 50.

A form of lupus that is confined to the skin is the discoid variant. Discoid lupus primarily involves the scalp, face, and ears and often begins as reddened, inflamed patches, which, over time, develop into discolored scars. Scalp involvement may result in permanent hair loss. Conversion of discoid lupus to the systemic form is rare.

As SLE may involve many organ systems, a coordinated multispecialty medical approach to management is prudent. Lesions of discoid lupus may respond to topical and intralesional steroids and are best managed by a dermatologist.

SCLERODERMA

Scleroderma is an uncommon skin condition characterized by hardening (fibrosis) of the skin and connective tissues. Fibrosis is triggered by the abnormal production and accumulation of collagen. The most serious form, called systemic sclerosis, can involve internal organs, such as the kidneys, heart, and lungs. Many patients experience an exaggerated response to cold, manifested as pain and color changes of the fingers. This is known as Raynaud's phenomenon. A localized form that affects only the skin is called morphea.

Systemic sclerosis, like lupus, merits evaluation by multiple medical specialists. Morphea is best managed by a dermatologist.

DERMATOMYOSITIS

Dermatomyositis is a progressive autoimmune disorder marked by inflammation and degeneration of muscle tissue. This leads to aches and profound weakness. The characteristic skin finding is a reddish-purple discoloration localized to the eyelids, cheeks, and nasal bridge (heliotrope rash). Papules may also arise on the knuckles (Gottron's sign). Most cases respond to high-dose oral steroid therapy. As with lupus, affected individuals are urged to apply broad-spectrum sunscreen and wear protective clothing when outdoors.

25

Sports and Skin

ATHLETES ARE PRONE TO A NUMBER OF SKIN CONDITIONS, SOME TRIVIAL and others not so. Fungi, yeast, and bacteria flourish in moist environments. Sweaty clothing helps promote growth of these microorganisms. Fungal spores shed from an individual with athlete's foot may be spread from the floor of a damp locker room. Plantar warts (caused by a virus) are transmitted in similar fashion. Acne may be worsened by sporting activities that involve heat, pressure, and occlusion. Appropriately named acne mechanica occurs under helmets and shoulder pads of football and hockey players.

Direct trauma can also affect the skin. Getting hit in the thigh with a line-drive baseball will, of course, result in a bruise. Constant rubbing of a sneaker against the foot will create a friction blister. Friction from clothing and tight bras may result in irritation and even bleeding of the nipples (so-called jogger's nipples). Tennis toe (subungual hematoma) is a painful traumatic condition caused by blood accumulation under the nail. Draining the trapped fluid provides immediate relief.

Of course, outside temperature alone can directly affect the skin. On cold winter days, one should wear layers of nonrestrictive clothing to prevent frostbite, paying attention to adequately protect the ears, nose, fingers, and toes. Very hot weather contributes to overheating, which can induce fluid loss and dehydration.

Swimmer's ear (otitis externa) is an infection of the outer ear canal. Children and teenagers who spend ample time in water are prone to this condition. Itching and pain are the main symptoms, and most cases will

129

respond to topical antibacterial ear drops. Swimmer's itch is a completely different entity and is caused by a parasite that ordinarily affects birds and snails but can also burrow through the skin of humans. The parasite quickly dies but induces an allergic reaction. Children are most often affected when swimming or wading in infested water. The disorder is quite benign, and the itchy rash will resolve spontaneously in a few days.

From a skin standpoint, wrestling—being an extreme, unprotected contact sport—is fraught with danger. Bacteria that cause impetigo and viruses that cause molluscum contagiosum are readily transmitted from person to person.

Some conditions have even been assigned wrestling nomenclature. Tinea gladiatorum is a fungal infection that affects wrestlers. The disorder is classic ringworm (tinea corporis), with individual lesions manifesting redness and scaling. Extensive cases are best treated with oral antifungal therapy.

More serious is herpes gladiatorum, a herpes simplex viral infection occurring in wrestlers. The blistering lesions cause pain and may be accompanied by fever, chills, fatigue, and swollen glands. As is common with other infections in athletes, herpes is spread by skin-to-skin contact. The condition is treated with oral antiviral medications.

The CDC first warned two decades ago of an increasing number of competitive athletes diagnosed with the antibiotic-resistant staph infection MRSA. MRSA, which can resemble an ordinary boil, may be passed to other players by skin-to-skin contact. Multiple cases have been documented in wrestlers and football players, but even fencers, cross-country runners, and field hockey players are at risk. Contributory factors include shared facilities and equipment and poor hygiene. The CDC recommends covering all wounds, thoroughly cleaning all shared equipment on a regular basis, and washing hands at frequent intervals.

26

Skin of Color

SKIN OF COLOR CONSTITUTES A WIDE RANGE OF ETHNICITIES AND RACES, including African Americans, Hispanics, and Asians. By 2050, persons of color will comprise at least half of the US population. And darker skin types are more prone to a variety of skin conditions.

Postinflammatory hyperpigmentation (PIH) is the name given to skin darkening that results secondary to trauma, such as a scratch, or from inflammatory skin disorders, such as acne. Acne is the most frequently encountered skin condition in African Americans and is the second most common skin problem in Asians. In darker skin, color changes induced by inflammation may persist and prove cosmetically unacceptable. Topical retinoids (chapter 16) are helpful in preventing acne and may lighten darkened areas as well. Compounds containing the substance hydroquinone may also be effective. Sunscreen is advised for daytime use, as sunlight can darken preexisting discolored areas.

Hidradenitis is a chronic inflammatory condition localized to the underarms, groin, and backside. The disease manifests as boils that are painful and drain pus. Blacks have an incidence three times higher than whites. Treatment with oral antibiotics is a mainstay of therapy, although surgical intervention is required at times. Two injectable drugs, Humira and Cosentyx, are approved as therapy.

Vitiligo is the result of pigment loss. Although this condition occurs in equal frequency among all racial and ethnic groups, the consequences

131

are much more apparent in darker-skinned individuals. Repigmentation of widespread disease is difficult.

Exaggerated scars called keloids may arise secondary to small abrasions, surgical wounds, or ear piercing. Some keloids form from pimples, especially when arising on the chest, back, or neck. Keloids are most common in black skin and are unsightly and, at times, painful. Injection of a steroid solution into the keloid can result in shrinkage. Surgical excision is also an option, although the recurrence rate may be as high as 75 percent.

Razor bumps are also more common in African Americans. Black hair is distinguished by curved hair shafts. Following a close shave, newly emerging pointed hairs turn downward and pierce the surface of the skin, resulting in irritation and bumps. This condition is called pseudofolliculitis barbae, and it affects approximately 50 percent of black men. Growing a beard results in cure; as the hair lengthens, it lifts out of the skin. Use of a special straight razor or an electric razor may prevent recurrence. Electrolysis and laser hair removal are therapeutic options that require multiple treatment sessions.

Skin cancer is less common in black individuals, as pigment protects against the damaging effects of sunlight. However, darker-skinned persons are not immune and should be especially vigilant for pigment changes affecting the palms, the soles, and beneath the nails. These are the most common sites for melanoma, which can be deadly if not diagnosed early.

Persons of Hispanic origin are the second-largest racial and ethnic group and are the principal driver of US population growth. Skin coloration varies greatly and ranges from lighter to darker complexions. Those with darker skin are more prone to melasma, a facial pigmentation affecting the cheeks, upper lip, and forehead of females. As exposure to sunlight worsens the condition, use of a high-SPF sunscreen is essential to prevent further darkening. Darkened areas may also result from acne warranting aggressive treatment. The incidence of skin cancer is increasing in Latinos, and the rate of melanoma has risen 20 percent over the past two decades.

27

Skin First Aid

BURNS

Burns may be caused by thermal, chemical, radioactive, or electrical agents. Burns are usually classified into the following three types:

- A first-degree burn involves only the outermost layers of the epidermis and results in swollen red skin that is tender and painful. This type of burn rapidly heals within one to two weeks without scarring. Examples of a first-degree burn include a moderate to severe sunburn or a burn resulting from a low-intensity heat source.
- A second-degree burn extends below the epidermis to the dermis but does not involve deeper structures, such as hair follicles. Second-degree burns are characterized by painful blisters and marked swelling. If left undisturbed, the skin heals within two to three weeks, again without scarring. Brief exposure to a hot liquid or curling iron might result in a second-degree burn.
- A third-degree burn destroys both the epidermis and the dermis. Because nerve endings are destroyed, severe pain is uncommon. Blistering, a function of dermal swelling, does not occur. Healing is slow, and scarring is anticipated. Skin grafting may be required.

Superficial burns can be managed without the intervention of a physician. Immediately following a burn, apply cold packs or ice to the burned area, or immerse the region in cold tap water. Coldness relieves pain, reduces swelling, and limits the extent of damage. Best results are achieved if such therapy is instituted within one hour after injury. Trivial burns require no dressings or medications. If the skin is broken, application of a topical antibiotic is recommended.

The initial treatment of a chemical burn entails immediate and thorough irrigation with water. Dependent on the chemicals involved, two to four hours of continuous washing may be required to limit the depth of injury. Neither chemical nor electrical burns are appropriate for self-care, and physician consultation should be sought as soon as possible.

Persons with burns of more than minor extent should be treated in a hospital emergency room, where removal of injured tissue (debridement) may be necessary.

INSECTS AND THE SKIN

Most humans tolerate insects to a remarkable degree. Tolerance rapidly dissipates when insects start to feed on our skin or terrorize us with their stingers. Several types of insects frequently abuse human flesh.

Bees

Bees pollinate flowers and manufacture honey. Occasionally, a nasty one will sting. Bee and wasp stings are painful and cause immediate swelling and redness. Wasps and bumblebees do not leave stingers behind and can therefore sting repeatedly. The stinger of the honeybee commonly breaks off within the skin, resulting in the insect's death.

If stung, flick the insect off, and do not squeeze it. Should the stinger remain, carefully remove it with tweezers. Cold compresses or ice applied at the sting site may lessen the severity of the reaction. Calamine lotion or a medicated steroid cream may also afford some relief.

Allergy to bee venom occurs in less than 1 percent of the population. Those affected experience serious, life-threatening reactions when stung. Symptoms of generalized allergy include tongue and throat swelling, dizziness, and difficulty breathing. As most deaths occur within thirty minutes of a sting, sensitive persons should carry an epinephrine injector (EpiPen) whenever outdoors in temperate weather. An allergist can administer desensitization injections to diminish the severity and danger of bee stings.

Mosquitoes

The ordinary mosquito bite produces an elevated bump that itches. A localized bite requires no treatment, although calamine lotion or cortisone cream may lessen the itching. In the tropics, mosquitoes transmit serious diseases, including yellow fever and malaria. In the United States, mosquitoes were generally thought to be mere nuisances until the recognition of the West Nile virus in 1999. Although infection is usually asymptomatic, about 20 percent of patients will develop flu-like symptoms shortly after being bit by an infected mosquito, and about 1 in 150 will experience severe neurologic disease, which can result in coma and lifelong disability. Mosquitoes also transmit Eastern equine encephalitis, which may be fatal. Locally acquired mosquito-transmitted malaria infection is rare in the United States and has most recently been reported in Florida.

In areas where mosquito disease spread has been identified, vigorous eradication endeavors are often initiated. Wearing hats and long-sleeved clothing is of benefit. The gold standard of insect repellants is DEET, which is certified as safe by the Environmental Protection Agency. Concentrations ranging from 20 to 25 percent are found in several topical preparations. Alternatives to DEET are picaridin and oil of lemon eucalyptus.

Spiders

Most spider bites cause minor swelling, redness, pain, or itching. Application of ice eases the discomfort, and a corticosteroid cream will minimize redness and itching.

The two spiders that cause serious reactions in the United States are the black widow and the brown recluse. The black widow commonly nests in cellars, outhouses, and sheds. The dangerous female is recognized by a reddish-orange hourglass configuration on its belly. Chills, vomiting, and cramps develop minutes after a bite. Fortunately, these bites are rarely fatal.

The brown recluse spider is widely distributed in the central and southern United States. This is a small dark brown creature with a characteristic violin-shaped mark on its head. The spider hides in closets and drawers. A bite is often followed several hours later by intense local pain and swelling. In severe cases, the affected area turns black, and gangrene may ensue. Most bites warrant medical evaluation.

Ticks

Ticks suck human blood. Once on the body, a tick surreptitiously inserts its head under the skin and engages in its vampire-like activities. Undetected, a tick may remain at this site for days.

Ticks should be removed with care, firmly grasped with tweezers and slowly withdrawn from the body. A tick should never be forcibly removed, because the head will remain under the skin, leading to a slow-healing sore. Following tick removal, wash the affected area with soap, and apply an antibiotic ointment.

Ticks spread Rocky Mountain spotted fever, a serious disease with a high fatality rate. For this reason, anyone recently bitten by a tick who develops sudden fever, headache, or skin eruption should seek emergency medical consultation.

Ticks also spread Lyme disease, a condition often accompanied by a circular red rash. Nearly half a million new cases occur in the United States each year. Untreated, Lyme disease may result in crippling arthritis.

Fleas

Fleas are an embarrassing problem, not so much to dogs and cats but to people. These tiny, wingless, bloodthirsty insects often cause intensely itchy red bumps. Approximately 50 percent of the population are not sensitive (allergic), so a pet owner may become aware of the problem only after other family members begin to itch. Scratching bites may lead to open areas and infection.

Ridding one's pet of fleas is no easy task. Flea collars are the most popular but probably least effective means of pet treatment. Flea soaps, shampoos, and pills can kill adult fleas on animals but do not provide lasting protection against reinfection. Thorough cleaning and vacuuming, including carpets and pet bedding, along with a pesticide spray, are necessary steps to flea-proof an infested house. The itch of fleabites will be diminished by application of topical steroids. More extensive cases may warrant oral steroid therapy.

Chiggers

Chiggers are tiny reddish-hued mites that are difficult to see without a magnifying glass. Unlike ticks, they do not burrow but attach themselves to the skin and inject saliva containing digestive enzymes. This process induces irritation and severe itching some twelve to twenty-four hours later. Raised reddened welts appear at the site, and these may last up to two weeks. Preferred areas are the ankles, the armpits, the belt line, and other skin folds. Chiggers, fortunately, do not transmit disease, but their bites can become secondarily infected.

Chiggers prefer warm weather and become inactive when the temperature falls below 60 degrees. They live in grass and foliage. As they do not burrow under the skin, simply rubbing affected areas or bathing suffices to remove the critters. DEET application will dissuade chiggers from crawling onto the skin.

DOG, CAT, AND HUMAN BITES

At times, wildlife—certain people included—bite. Any bite that punctures the skin surface warrants medical attention. Each year, more than two million bites are reported, with dogs being responsible for some 85 percent of these cases. One-third of all animal bites occur in children, and about one-half of all bites are considered provoked. Bites account for about 1 percent of all emergency room visits. Approximately 1 percent of dog bites and 6 percent of cat bites result in admission to a hospital.

Dog jaws are powerful and may induce crush injury, lacerations, and puncture wounds. Cat bites are usually of the puncture variety. Cat bites are three times more likely to become infected, as cats carry more dangerous germs in their saliva. All animal bites should be cleansed thoroughly with soap and water as soon as possible. Bleeding is best controlled by application of pressure. If the wound is swollen, apply ice wrapped in a towel. Obtain a history of rabies vaccination from the owner. If the owner is unknown, attempt to keep the animal in sight until animal control personnel arrive.

A cat bite or scratch can lead to cat scratch fever disease, which is caused by a bacterium. The condition begins as a reddened pimple at the site of injury, followed by painful, swollen glands and flu-like symptoms. Most cases are self-limited and resolve without treatment, although antibiotic therapy will shorten the duration.

Human bites too may prove serious, as the mouth is a reservoir for some nasty germs. Approximately 250,000 human bites are reported each year.

Some occur as a result of fighting; others occur while playing. Regardless, any human bite that breaks the skin surface should be copiously cleansed with soap and water and monitored for signs of infection. Because of the potential for serious infection, many physicians will institute a three- to seven-day course of prophylactic antibiotic therapy.

Conclusion

Your skin—bruised, bitten, and blistered. From bites to solar radiation, frigid blasts to searing heat, this resilient organ takes quite a beating. It's molested by the environment, feasted on by teeming hordes of invisible microbes, and subtly traumatized on a daily basis. No wonder skin occasionally displays wear and tear.

In the search for longevity and lasting beauty, a good starting point is indeed your outermost cover. Be kind to your skin. It just may last a lifetime!

About the Author

DR. STEPHEN M. SCHLEICHER brings three decades of experience in the field of dermatology. He graduated Phi Beta Kappa from Rutgers University, received his medical degree with academic honors from the Drexel/Hahnemann Medical College, and completed his dermatology residency at the Temple Skin and Cancer Hospital. The author of three books and hundreds of journal case reports, Dr. Schleicher served for ten years on the advisory board of the Day Spa Association and the editorial board of the journal *Emergency Medicine*. He cohosted both the radio call-in show *Speaking of Your Skin* and the cable television show *Skin Sense*. He also cofounded the first joint podiatry and dermatology fellowship in the United States.

The dermatologist founder and director of the DermDox Dermatology Centers, PC (dermdoxcenters.com), Dr. Schleicher has served as a principal investigator for more than fifty phase I–IV clinical trials. He is a pioneer in the field of teledermatology, and his weekly column (DermDx) in the journal *Clinical Advisor* is viewed by thousands of medical practitioners. He is a past Computerworld honors laureate and recipient of the Outstanding Specialty Provider award by the nonprofit Volunteers in Medicine. Dr. Schleicher provides clinical instruction in dermatology to physician assistant students enrolled at King's College and Misericordia and Arcadia universities.

Index

American Vitiligo Research
    Foundation, 42
Amnesteem, 85
Amzeeq (minocycline), 84
anal itching (pruritus ani), 20–21
anaphylaxis, 121
ancillary treatments (for acne), 86
androgenetic alopecia, 59–60
antiaging compounds, 24–25
antiandrogen, 85
antibacterials
    azelaic acid, 84
    benzoyl peroxide, 82
    for treatment of boils, 111
    for treatment of eczema, 93
    for treatment of impetigo, 109
    for treatment of intertrigo, 108
    for treatment of swimmer's ear,
        129–130
    zinc, 15
antibiotics
    clindamycin, 82
    for treatment of acne, 84
    for treatment of boils, 111
    for treatment of burns, 134
    for treatment of cat bites, 138
    for treatment of cellulitis, 109
    for treatment of hidradenitis, 131
    for treatment of hives, 123
    for treatment of human bites, 139
    for treatment of impetigo, 109
    for treatment of Lyme disease, 112
    for treatment of MRSA, 111
    for treatment of necrotizing
        fasciitis, 110

for treatment of perioral
    dermatitis, 90
for treatment of populopustular
    rosacea, 89
for treatment of severe sunburn, 31
for treatment of ticks, 136
for treatment of yeast vaginitis, 107
antifungals
    FDA approval of, 67–68
    for treatment of athlete's foot, 105
    for treatment of seborrheic
        dermatitis, 65
    for treatment of tina
        gladiatorum, 130
    for treatment of tinea cruris, 106
    for treatment of tinea
        versicolor, 107
    for treatment of yeast vaginitis, 107
antihistamines
    for treatment of atopic
        dermatitis, 93
    for treatment of bedbugs, 121
    for treatment of hives, 123
antioxidants, 5, 7, 8, 9, 10, 11, 13, 14, 15
antiperspirants, 75, 76
antiviral medications
    for treatment of herpes, 114
    for treatment of herpes
        gladiatorum, 130
    for treatment of HIV, 118
    for treatment of shingles, 115
anti-yeast creams, for treatment of
    intertrigo, 108
apremilast (Otezla), 102
Apretude, 118
Aquanil, 95

Aquaphor, 92

Arazlo (tazarotene), 83

asorbic acid (vitamin C), 13, 15, 25, 44

astringents, 81, 89

Atarax (hydroxyzine), 122

athletes, skin conditions of, 129–130

athlete's foot (tinea pedis), 105

atopic dermatitis (eczema), 20, 91–93

Atralin (tretinoin), 83

autoimmune diseases

    dermatomyositis, 128

    lupus, 127

    scleroderma, 128

Avage, 24

Avar, 83, 89

Aveeno, 92

avobenzone (Parsol 1789), 33

Avodart (dutasterid), 57, 59, 60

azelaic acid (Azelex, Finacea), 44, 84, 89

B

baby soap, 95

bacterial infections, 109–112

Barbie drug (AKA melatonin-2), 41

baricitinib (Olumiant), 61

basal cell carcinoma, 52–53

bedbugs, 121

bees, treatment for stings from, 134

Bellafill, 28

Belotero, 27

Benadryl (diphenhydramine), 122

BenzaClin (clindamycin), 83, 84

benzoyl peroxide, 81, 82–83, 84, 87, 89

berdazimer (Zelsuvmi), 116

beta-carotene, 12

betamethasone (Diprolene), 100

bimatoprost (Latisse), 60

Bimzelx (bimekizumab), 102

biologics, 68, 101, 102, 123

biotin, 6–7, 66

birthmarks, 46

bites

    from dogs, cats, and humans,
        138–139

    from insects, 134–138

black widow spider, 136

blackheads, 78–79, 86

bleaching, as treatment for objectionable
    hairs, 64

blond hair, 56

blood vessels (venules), dilation of,
    72–74

blue light sources, for treatment of
    acne, 86

blush zone, 88

body dissatisfaction, causes of, 40

body lice, 120

body weight, effect of on skin, 4–5

boils, 110–111

botanicals, 5, 6

Botox, 26–27, 77

botulinum neurotoxins, 77

Brella, 77

brimonidine (Mirvaso), 89

British Journal of Dermatology, on use of
    sunscreen, 34

broad spectrum sunscreens, 33

brodalumab (Siliq), 102

brown recluse spider, 136

bruising, 74–75

burns, first aid for, 133–134

butyl stearate, 18

C

calamine lotion, 134

calcineurin inhibitors, 42

calluses, 48–49

candidiasis, 107

cannabidiol (CBD), 7

cantharidin, 115

canthaxanthin, 37

carbohydrates, contributions of to
healthy skin, 4

carotenoids, 10

cellulite, 2, 69–70

cellulitis, 109–110

Centers for Disease Control (CDC)
on cause of melanomas, 53
on genital herpes, 113
on HPV vaccination, 48
on MRSA in athletes, 130
on syphilis, 112

CeraVe, 92, 95

Certain Dri, 76

certolizumab (Cimzia), 101

cervical cancer, genital warts and, 48

Cetaphil, 92, 95

cetirizine (Zyrtec), 122

chemical peels, 25–26, 44

cherry angiomas, 72–73

chicken pox, 114–115, 116, 117

chiggers, treatment and prevention
from, 137–138

chloasma ("the mask of pregnancy"), 43

choline, 9

chronological aging, 23

Cibinqo (abrocitnib), 93

ciclopirox (Penlac), 68, 106

Cimzia (certolizumab), 101

Claravis, 85

Claritin (loratadine), 122

clascoterone (Winlevi), 85

Clean and Clear, 83

Cleocin T, 84

clindamycin (Acanya, BenzaClin, Duac,
Onexton), 83, 84

clobetasol (Impoyz, Temovate), 42, 100

closed comedones, 78–79

Clostridium histolyticum, 70

clotrimazole (Lotrimin), 105

clotrimazole troches (Mycelex), 108

clubbed nails, 66

coconut oil, 8

coenzyme Q10 (ubiquinone-10), 7

coffeeberry extract, 8

cold sores, 113

collagen
effects of aging on, 22
as one of the foundations of
dermis, 27
production of, 10, 13, 87

comedones (whiteheads and
blackheads), 78–79

common wart, 47

compression stockings, 74

Condylox (podofilox gel), 48

congenital syphilis, 112

contact dermatitis, 19, 96

contraceptives, for treatment of acne,
84–85

Coolibar, 33

Coppertone QT (Quick Tanning), 36

corns, 48–49

corticosteroids, 136

Cosentyx (secukinumab), 102, 131
cosmetics, allergic reactions from,
    95–96
Covermark, 43
crab lice, 120
crisaborole (Eucrisa), 92–93
cryosurgery (liquid nitrogen), 44, 46,
    48, 51, 53, 115
curcumin, 12
cyclosporine, 93, 100, 101
cystatin, 107–108
cysts, associated with acne, 78, 79

D

dandruff (seborrheic dermatitis), 15,
    64–65
dapsone gel (Aczone), 84
Daxxify, 26
DEET, 112, 135, 138
Degree Invisible Solid, 76
delusions of parasitosis, 20
Demodex, 89
deodorants, 75
Department of Health and Human
    Services (US), on ultraviolet
    light, 36
depigmentation, 42, 43
depilatory creams, 64
Depo-Provera, hirsutism and, 63
Dermablend, 43
dermabrasion, 87
dermal fillers, 27–28
dermatitis
    allergic dermatitis, 98
    atopic dermatitis (eczema), 20,
        91–93

contact dermatitis, 19, 96
dermatitis herpetiformis, 4
irritant dermatitis, 94–95
plant dermatitis, 97–98
seborrheic dermatitis, 15, 64–
    65, 118
dermatomyositis, 128
dermis, 1–2
Descovy, 118
Dexenex, 105
DHS, 100
DHS Tar, 65
DHS Zinc (zinc pyrithione), 65
diabetes, 123–124
Dial, 111
diclofenac (Solaraze), 51
diet, role of in skin conditions, 4
Differin (adapalene), 44, 71, 83
Diflucan (fluconazole), 107, 108
dihydroxyacetone (DHA), 36–37, 43
Dilantin, hirsutism and, 63
dimethyl sulfoxide (DMSO), 114
dimethylglyoxime, 97
diphenhydramine (Benadryl), 122
Diprolene (betamethasone), 100
discoid lupus, 127
dishpan hands, 94
Ditropan (oxybutynin), 76
Doryx (doxycycline), 84, 89
Dove Invisible Solid, 76
Dovonex, 100
doxycycline (Acticlate, Doryx), 84, 89
Drionic (iontophoresis) therapy, 76
drospirenone and ethinyl estradiol
    (Yaz), 85
dry skin (xerosis)

of excimer laser, 100
of Ilumya, 102
of isotretinoin, 85
of Jublia, 67
of Kerydin, 67
of Klisyri, 51
of Litfulo, 61
of Mirvaso, 89
of Olumiant, 61
of Opzelura, 43, 92
of oral tranexamic acid, 44
of Ortho Tri-Cyclen, 85
of Otezla, 102
of Penlac, 68
of Propecia, 57–58
of Refissa, 24
of Restylane, 27
of Rhofade, 89
of Rinvoq, 93
of Rogaine, 57
of Skyrizi, 102
of Solaraze, 51
of Soolantra, 89
of Sotyktu, 102
of Stelara, 102
of Taltz, 102
of tazarotene, 12
of Tazorac, 100
of TNF alpha inhibitors,
    101–102
of Tremfya, 102
of tretinoin, 12
of Vtama, 93, 100
of Winlevi, 85
of Xolair, 122
of Yaz, 85

of Ycanth, 115–116
of Zelsuvmi, 116
of Zoryve, 65, 100
on electrolysis, 64
on hair removal devices, 63
on hair-smoothing and
    straightening products, 62
on indoor tanning, 35
on products approved to slow down
    or reverse male pattern
    alopecia, 57–58
on sun protection factor rating
    (SPF), 34
on use of canthaxanthin, 37
on use of DHA, 37
on use of indoor tan spraying, 37
on use of neurotoxins, 26
on use of over-the-counter bleach
    creams, 44
on use of spray-on sunscreens, 35
on use of tranexamic acid, 44
on use of tyrosine, 37
warning about high-dose biotin,
    7, 66
warnings about Cibinqo and
    Rinvoq, 93
female pattern hair loss (androgenetic
    alopecia), 59–60
fever blisters, 113
fexofenadine (Allegra), 122
fibrosis, 128
Finacea (azelaic acid), 44, 84, 89
finasteride (Propecia), 57, 58–59
first aid (for skin), 133–139
flat wart, 47
flavonoids, 11

fleas, treatment and prevention
from, 137
flesh-eating bacteria (necrotizing
fasciitis), 110
fluconazole (Diflucan), 107, 108
fluorouracil, 51, 53
folliculitis, 63
food, allergic reactions from, 4
fractional photothermolysis, 71
fungal infections, 104–107

G

Gardasil 9 vaccine, 48
genital herpes, 113–114
genital wart, 47, 48
German measles, 116
Gloves in a Bottle, 95
glycolic acid, 25, 44
glycopyrronium (Robinul), 76
glycosaminoglycan, 9
goose bumps, 55
Gottron's sign, 128
grape seed extract, 8
gray hair, 56
griseofulvin, 105
growth factors, 9
guselkumab (Tremfya), 102

H

hair
damage to, 56–57
differences in among races, 56
excess of (hirsutism), 62–63
gray hair, 56
growth of scalp hair, 55
loss of, 57–62

myths about, 62
normal hair, 55
removal of unwanted hair, 63–64
split ends, 56–57
hair products, for hair-smoothing and
straightening, 62
hair transplantation, 59, 60
halobetasol (Halog), 100
Harvard University, study of use of
vitamin D, 14
Head & Shoulders (selenium sulfide),
65, 107
heliotrope rash, 128
herald patch, 117
heredity
as factor contributing to skin
aging, 23
role of in acne, 79
role of in atopic dermatitis, 92
role of in psoriasis, 99
role of in severity of cellulite, 69
role of in skin cancer, 50
herpes gladiatorum, 130
herpes simplex, 113–114
herpes zoster (shingles), 114–115
hidradenitis, 131
hirsutism, 62–63
HIV, 118
hives (urticaria), 121
hormonal agents, for treatment of acne,
84–85
hormones, role in development of acne,
79, 80
hot-comb alopecia, 62
humectants, 18
Humira (adalimumab), 101, 131

kinetin, 9
Klaron, 83, 89
Klisyri (tirbanibulin), 51

L

Lamisil (terbinafine), 67, 105
lanolin, 18
laser
  ablative laser resurfacing, 28–29
  for correction of scarring from
    acne, 87
  excimer laser, 100
  nonablative laser resurfacing, 28, 29
  pulsed dye laser (PDL), 72
  removal of unwanted hair with,
    63, 64
  removal of warts with, 48
  for treatment of acne, 86
  for treatment of fungal nail
    infections, 68
  for treatment of leg veins, 73
  for treatment of stretch marks, 71
  for treatment/improvement of
    cellulite, 70
laser rejuvenation, 28–29
latex, allergic reactions from, 98
Latisse (bimatoprost), 60
lecithin, 9
leg veins, 73–74
lentigo maligna (Hutchinson's freckle),
  51, 52
leukoplakia, 51, 52, 53
Levicyn, 93
lice, 120
lichenification, 91
lip augmentation, 28

liquid nitrogen (cryosurgery), 44, 46,
  48, 51, 53, 115
Litfulo (ritlecitinib), 61
liver spots, 44
looks, preoccupation with, 40
looksmaxing, use of term, 40
loratadine (Claritin), 122
Lotrimin (clotrimazole), 105
lycopene, 10
Lyme disease, 111, 137
lysine pills, 114

M

male pattern baldness, 57–59
malignant melanoma, 53–54
marionette lines, 28
"the mask of pregnancy" (chloasma), 43
massage, for treatment of stretch
  marks, 70
measles, 116
melanin, 3, 37, 56
melanocytes, 3
melanoma, 35, 53–54, 132
melasma, 43–44, 132
melatonin-2, 37, 41
mesotherapy, 9
methicillin-resistant staphylococcus
  aureus (MRSA), 111
methotrexate, 93, 100, 101
metronidazole (Metrogel, Moritate),
  89, 90
Mexoryl SX (terephthalylidene
  dicamphor sulfonic acid), 33
miconazole (Micatin), 105
microdermabrasion, 25, 44
microneedling, 87

minerals, 5

minocycline (Amzeeq, Minocin, Solodyn), 84

minoxidil (Rogaine), 57, 58, 59–60

MiraDry system, 76–77

Mirvaso (brimonidine), 89

moisturizers

    acne and, 80

    aloe vera as ingredient in, 6

    with sunscreen, 24

    for treatment of dry skin, 18

    for treatment of eczema, 92

    for treatment of stretch marks, 70

moles, 46

molluscum contagiosum, 115–116, 130

moniliasis, 107

monobenzone, 43

Morgellons disease, 20

Moritate (metronidazole), 89, 90

morphea, 128

mosquitoes, treatment and prevention from, 135

MRSA (methicillin-resistant staphylococcus aureus), 111

mupirocin, 109

Mycelex (clotrimazole troches), 108

Myorisan, 85

N

nails

    acrylic nails, 67

    brittle nails, 66

    deformities of, 66

    described, 65

    growth of, 65–66

    infections of, 67, 106

    length of, 67

nasolabial folds, 28

National Alopecia Areata Foundation, 61

National Psoriasis Foundation

    study of psoriasis patients, 99

    website, 103

necrosis (skin breakdown), 28

necrotizing fasciitis (flesh-eating bacteria), 110

Neoral, 101

neurotixins, 26

Neutrogena T/Gel, 65

nevus/nevi, 46–47

niacinamide, 10

nickel allergy, 97

nicotinamide (vitamin B3), 10, 51

Nix, 120

Nizoral (ketoconazole), 65, 107

nonablative laser resurfacing, 28, 29

nummular eczema, 91

nutraceuticals, 5

O

ocular rosacea, 88

oil (sebaceous) glands. See sebaceous (oil) glands

ointments

    antibacterial ointments, 109

    antibiotic ointments, 136

    antiviral ointments, 114

    green-tea ointment, 11

    steroid ointments, 92, 100

    for treatment of brittle nails, 66

    for treatment of dry skin, 18

    for treatment of eczema, 92

Protopic (tacrolimus), 42, 92, 93
PRP (platelet-rich plasma), 27, 60
pruritus, 19
pruritus ani (anal itching), 20–21
pseudofolliculitis barbae, 132
Pseudomonas, 66
psoriasis, 68, 99–103
psoriatic arthritis, 102
ptosis, 26
pulsed dye laser (PDL), 72
pustules, associated with acne, 78, 79
pychogenol, 11

Q

Qbrexza, 76
Quick Tanning (Coppertone QT), 36

R

radiation therapy, 53
Radiesse, 28
Raynaud's phenomenon, 128
razor bumps, 132
red hair, 56
red light sources, for treatment of
    acne, 86

S

Sabtreo, 83
SAD (seasonal affective disorder),
    37–38
Safeguard, 111
salicylic acid, 25, 81, 87
Sandimmune, 101
sarecycline (Seysara), 84
scabies, 119–120

Refissa, 24
Remicade (infliximab), 101
repigmentation, 56, 132
Restylane, 27
resveratrol, 8, 25
Retin-A, 24, 71, 83
retinoids, 9, 24, 71, 83, 84, 87, 100, 131
retinol, 12, 25
retinyl palmitate, 12
Revanesse Versa, 27
Rezamid, 83
RHA collection (RHA 2, RHA 3, RHA
    4), 27
rhinophyma, 88
Rhofade (oxymetazoline), 89
Rid, 120
Rinvoq (upadacitinib), 93
risankizumab (Skyrizi), 102
Rit SunGuard, 33
ritlecitinib (Litfulo), 61
Robinul (glycopyrronium), 76
Rocky Mountain spotted fever, 136
roflumilast (Zorvye), 65, 100
Rogaine (minoxidil), 57, 58, 59–60
rosacea, 88–90
ruxolitinib (Opzelura), 42–43, 92

scars
    associated with acne, 78, 79, 81, 85
    associated with boils, 110
    associated with burns, 133
    associated with lupus, 127
    associated with skin of color, 132
    cannabidiol for treatment of, 7

social media, as source of medical information, 40
sodium tetradecyl sulfate, 73
solar keratosis (actinic keratosis), 10, 51, 53
Solaraze (diclofenac), 51
Solodyn (minocycline), 84
Solumbra, 33
Soolantra, 89
Soriatane (acitretin), 100–101
Sotret, 85
Sotyku, 102
soy proteins, 11
SPF (sun protection factor rating), 34, 38, 44, 127, 132
spider veins, 72, 73
spiders, treatment for bites from, 136
spironolactone, 60
split ends, 56–57
spoon-shaped nails, 66
sports, and skin, 129–130
spot therapy, for acne, 81
squamous cell carcinoma, 53
staphylococcal infections, 110
STD (sexually transmitted disease), genital warts as, 47
Stelara (ustekinumab), 102
steroids
    for gaining muscle mass, 70
    for treatment of acne, 86
    for treatment of alopecia areata, 61
    for treatment of bedbugs, 121
    for treatment of bee stings, 134
    for treatment of dermatomyositis, 128
    for treatment of eczema, 92

for treatment of flea bites, 137
for treatment of hives, 123
for treatment of irritant dermatitis, 95
for treatment of keloids, 132
for treatment of lupus, 128
for treatment of melasma, 44
for treatment of paronychias, 67
for treatment of perioral dermatitis, 90
for treatment of psoriasis, 100
for treatment of seborrheic dermatitis, 65
for treatment of vitiligo, 42
stretch marks (striae distensae), 8, 70–71
subcutaneous (of fat) tissue, 2
subungual hematoma (tennis toe), 129
Sulfacet-R, 89
sulfur, 83, 87
sun protection, 31–34. *See also* protective clothing
sun protection factor rating (SPF), 34, 38, 44, 127, 132
sunburn, 30–31, 32–33, 34, 36, 42, 43, 47, 53, 83, 133
sunless tanning products, 36–37
sunlight
    as factor contributing to skin aging, 23
    impact of on skin, 30–39
    role of in acne treatment, 81
sunscreens, 6, 18, 24, 33–36, 38, 43–44, 51, 89, 127, 128, 131, 132
suntan, 30, 32, 37. *See also* tanning
superfoods, 8

159

swimmer's ear (otitis externa), 129–130
swimmer's itch, 130
sympathectomy, 77
syphilis, 112
systemic lupus erythematosus (SLE),
  127, 128
systemic sclerosis, 128

T

tacrolimus (Protopic), 42, 92, 93
Taltz (ixekixumab), 102
tamoxifen, hirsutism and, 63
tan accelerators, 37
tanning. *See also* suntan
  indoor tanning, 31, 35, 36, 127
  oral tanning pills, 37, 41
  self-tanning agents, 43
tanorexia, 36
tapinarof (Vtama), 93, 100
tar (DHS Tar, Neutrogena T/Gel,
  Tarsum), 65, 100
tavaborole (Kerydin), 67
tazarotene (Arazlo, Tazorac), 12, 24, 44,
  83, 100
tea extracts, 11
telangiectasias, 72
telogen effluvium, 60–61
Temovate (clobetasol), 42, 100
tennis toe (subungual hematoma), 129
terbinafine (Lamisil), 67, 105
terephthalylidene dicamphor sulfonic
  acid (Mexoryl SX), 33
testosterone, acne and, 79, 82
tetracycline, 84, 107
T/Gel, 100
thrush (oral candidiasis), 107–108

thyroid disease, 125–126
ticks, treatment for, 136–137
tildrakizumad (Ilumya), 102
tinea
  tinea capitis, 104–105
  tinea corporis (body ringworm),
    105, 130
  tinea cruris (jock itch), 106
  tinea gladiatorum, 130
  tinea pedis (athlete's foot), 105
  tinea versicolor, 106–107
tirbanibulin (Klisyri), 51
tissue stabilized-guided subcision, 70
TNF alpha inhibitors, 101–102
tocopherol acetate, 15
traction alopecia, 62
tralokinumab (Adbry), 93
tranexamic acid, 44
transgender men, acne and, 79, 82
Tremfya (guselkumab), 102
tretinoin (Atralin, Retin-A), 12, 24, 44,
  71, 83
trichloroacetic acid, 25
trichotillomania, 61–62
trifarotene (Aklief), 71, 83
Tri-Luma, 44
Truvada, 118
turmeric, 12
Twyneo, 83
tyrosine, 37

U

ubiquinone-10 (coenzyme Q10), 7
ugly duckling sign, 53
Ulesfia, 120
Ultra (Juvederm), 27

Printed in the United States
by Baker & Taylor Publisher Services

Printed in the United States
by Baker & Taylor Publisher Services